BRIEFINGS FROM A
DOCTOR'S
FOXHOLE

M. COLIN JORDAN

ACKNOWLEDGMENTS

With Love to My Wife Pamela Lahrs and to My Children Teresa, Angela, and Colin for Putting Up with Me

With Homage to My Mentors Ed Navarro, John D. Egan (Creighton University), Robert G. Petersdorf and Robert H. Williams (University of Washington), and Jack G. Stevens (University of California, Los Angeles)

Thanks for Review of the Manuscript by Pamela Lahrs, Bob Carlson, Kathy Ransdell, Richard E. Bryant, and Tom Bouse

Special Thanks to Bob Carlson for Rigorous and Vigorous Critique (All the Critique You Can Handle and Then Some)

ABOUT THE AUTHOR

M. Colin Jordan, MD is a university professor of internal medicine living with his wife Pamela in Oregon. He served as chief of infectious diseases for twenty-two years at the University of Minnesota Hospitals and Clinics in Minneapolis and at the Oregon Health & Science University in Portland. Earlier faculty appointments were at the University of California, Los Angeles (UCLA) and Davis. He has published over 200 scientific articles on infectious diseases and viruses, especially the herpes group, and he has an international reputation in his field. Dr. Jordan co-authored two editions of a textbook of infectious diseases (*Infectious Diseases: A Modern Treatise of Infectious Processes*) published by Lippincott in 1989 and 1994. *Briefings from a Doctor's Foxhole* is his first book written for the general reader.

NOTE TO READERS

Except for the author's mentors, the names of all patients and physicians in the book have been changed to preserve confidentiality.

CONTENTS

PROLOGUE

BRIEFINGS FROM A DOCTOR'S FOXHOLE

Maybe it all started that day I was born in a bomb shelter during the Blitz in industrial England. After the war, I was sure that once I got to blue collar America, I'd fit right in. On my first day at school, a mob laughed me out of the room, howling at a silly lad who talked funny wearing a shirt and tie, braces (suspenders), short pants, thick stockings to his knees, and a cap. Never mind. He'd be back tomorrow in trousers though he wasn't yet sixteen or eligible to wear them.

I wanted to be a doctor like our family doctor Ellen Hawkins with no idea how to go about it. My first mentor in the New World was a down-on-his-luck Native American minor league baseball pitcher who took me in stride when no one else had time. Fifteen years later, I was a doctor thanks to Ed Navarro and a college baseball scholarship.

The journey takes me to Seattle as an intern in the tumultuous '60s. While Vietnam rages on, so does the dreaded "doctor draft." Don't these damned wars ever end? Two weeks after they'd put MD next to my name, I take care of a young woman who nearly dies of an illegal septic abortion, six years before Roe v. Wade. I press on. Figuring out who's in my foxhole and who's not troubles me most. So it goes, more than thirty years in trenches mined by infectious diseases, where skirmishes between microbes and man play out everyday, and where lives are won or lost. I grapple with the drug culture, "the children of the sixties," survive a brutal residency, and investigate epidemics as an officer at the Centers for Disease Control. After I land a faculty position at the University Hospital in Los Angeles, the herpes virus research I love falters. Discouraged and bewildered, I nearly abandon what I see as "medicine's highest calling" for private practice. I muddle through a divorce and learn that my father, whom I thought had been killed on a D-Day beach, was now preaching fire and brimstone all over England. I could hardly wait to meet him.

Life and medicine are harsh, contentious now. Doctors harm patients, patients abuse doctors, doctors abuse themselves and their colleagues, and the litany of "bio-political crises" never ends. When that utter devastation called AIDS dawns in 1981, the landscape is forever changed. Doctors are now private detectives, sleazy voyeurs peering into bedrooms and bath houses, asking questions they don't want answered. Holier-than-thou vigilantes cluck their tongue and wag a finger until HIV infects heterosexuals, and "red-blooded American boys" start to catch it. Families want death certificates altered. Infected plasma donors wipe out a generation of hemophiliacs. About all doctors could do or say by then was to "go forth and sin no more." Aware of his own foibles, at least one doctor knows he'll never "practice" enough medicine to get it quite right. The reader may never see his or her physician in quite the same way again.

CHAPTER 1

A NAVAJO KNUCKLE CURVEBALL

"Hey, kid! Ya wanna pick up a couple a bucks helpin' me out in the garage?"

I knew who he was the second he hollered across the street. Sixty years later, he's still on my mind. Ed Navarro, a fiery American Indian, maybe too fiery, pitched for the Sacramento Solons in the Pacific Coast League. No one said "Native American" in those days. The Solons were the top farm team of the major league Boston Braves. On TV, Ed had a wicked curveball, a nasty moustache, and not enough "heat" to go with them. His fastball didn't have enough "giddy-up" on it.

He'd never make it to the big leagues ("the Bigs") even for "a cup a coffee" as they say in baseball parlance. Still twice, he was the man last cut when the Braves broke camp to end spring training. Biloxi, Lincoln, and Chattanooga had been his venues. I knew his grit, and I'd seen his fire. After we'd stacked up boxes and hung up tools in the garage, he asked me. "How old are you, son? You live around here?"

"I'm eleven, and I'm right where you found me, across the street. But I'm from England." Now, he knew what to expect.

"Yeah, you do talk kinda funny, like a kid I seen in the movies or on TV somewhere. How come you're in Southern California?"

"My dad was killed in France on D-Day. My mum met a GI later. So, I'm here." The story had always seemed a bit dodgy, but it was the one I had.

"Sorry to hear about your dad, but you could be somewhere a whole lot worse. Things OK at home?"

1

"I guess so, but they sure fight a lot."

After a smile and a nod, he wanted to talk about something else. "So, you were in England for the war?"

"Yeah, I was born in a bomb shelter, near Manchester. Jerry, - sorry, I mean the Germans - bombed us every night. The Nazis wanted to wipe out the factories in Coventry and Warrington that built the Spitfire and Hurricane fighter planes. Those planes and the Royal Air Force pilots were all we had to hold off the Luftwaffe."

Talk of the war always reminded me of my first day at school in America in 1947. I showed up for first grade wearing a shirt and tie, short pants and suspenders (braces, I called them), long stockings to my knees, and a little cap, a "Dickie." The kids laughed me out of the room, hooting and jeering. I ran home to my mother saying, "I can't go back without a proper pair of trousers," though I wasn't yet sixteen or eligible to wear them in the old country.

I cupped a palm over an eye to block the sun, squint up at him, and change the subject. I must have seemed like the precocious little shit I probably was, but here was my moment. "I've seen you pitch on TV. You're Ed Navarro, right?"

"You play ball?"

"I just tried out for Little League. Don't know yet if I made a team."

"What position do you play?"

"Second base and center field. I'm a lead-off hitter, and I pitch some."

"You pitch some? Now you're talkin.' Give me an hour or so to clean up around here and take a shower. Then ring the bell. Let's see what you got."

The West Coast didn't have major league ball in '52 and wouldn't until the Brooklyn Dodgers and New York Giants moved west in '58. Two minor league teams, the LA Angels and the Hollywood Stars, slugged it out. In Orange County, between LA and San Diego, I looked on as Gene Mauch, Steve Bilko, and Lee Walls hammered away on TV, hoping for a call-up to the Bigs.

Baseball's our great game, the game closest to life, and just about as cruel. I didn't know then that practicing medicine was much the same.

The best fail time and again and look feeble trying. The game will break your heart if you let it. To stay sane while watching, you need to be patient and hold on to your seat with both hands. Still, I loved the Brooklyn Dodgers, who lost to the New York Yankees any time they had a chance. Maybe that's why I loved them. I was an underdog kind of kid, and I never got over it.

———

An hour later, the neighbors heard horsehide whack on leather as we played ball in his front yard. He was burly in his T-shirt and jeans, though not as muscular as he'd looked in uniform on TV. He had some fat on him and a bit of a paunch to go with his macho. But his moustache was even more fantastic in real life.

"Hey, you're a ballplayer, kid! Let me grab a catcher's glove and have you pitch to me."

He squatted in position wearing a catcher's mask. I walked off the forty-four foot Little League pitching distance, fifteen of my longest strides, and turned to face him.

"OK. Let it go. Don't hold back. I can handle whatever you can throw."

I threw the first pitches in a measured kind of way, trying to hit his glove, wherever he put it, not sure how good a catcher he was. "You got great control, but can't you throw harder than that? You'll never get 'em out with that shit! Too much finesse. I know all about finesse, believe me. You got to intimidate the hitter. Come on! Let me have it. More heat. That's why we're here." No one had ever talked to me like this.

I let three pitches rip, hard as I could throw, puffing dust in all directions out of his mitt. "Wow, that's enough for me, son. What a fastball! You got more heat than I ever had." He grinned with an ease I'd never seen him show on TV. "Great stuff, I love the leverage you get off that back leg when you wind up. Maybe you'll play pro ball some day, kid."

I'd never be good enough for that. Besides, I wanted to be a doctor, like Ellen Hawkins, our family doctor. She was cool with kids and tough on parents as she flitted room to room in her white coat and half-spectacles. When she spoke to your mum and dad at the end of a visit, getting down to cases, she took off the glasses as if she were taking off the gloves. How much fun it was to see Dr. Hawkins give your parents hell over your lousy nutrition or neglected vaccinations! Maybe I'd never be good enough for that either.

"Kid, how come your legs are so strong?"

"I'm a dancer."

"A dancer? You're a dancer? "

"Yeah, you know. Tap, ballet, and acrobatic stuff."

"Ballet? You're kidding. You don't stand around all fagged out do you like those fruits on TV with their phony puffed-out crotches?"

"No, I've never seen them do that." I didn't tell him I'd seen gay young men with thunder in their thighs soar through the air and hoist ballerinas to the heavens.

"OK. I take your word on it. Come on over and set on the porch." His right hand caressed my shoulder as we ambled across the lawn. "Do you know anything about the knuckle curveball?"

"No, but you had a great curveball on TV. I loved the way it broke, and how the batters froze or whiffed at it! The announcers raved about that pitch."

"It was my meal ticket. I learned to throw it in Class A ball in Chattanooga. Josh Williams, a man from the Negro Leagues, taught me to throw it. He had major league stuff, the best pitcher I ever saw, and the only real pitching coach I ever had. But, you know, baseball didn't let Negroes into the majors until the great Jackie Robinson came up with Brooklyn in '47. Williams was a man, a father to me." He choked up a bit before going on. "You got a great arm, kid. I can teach you the knuckle curve if you want to throw it."

I didn't know what to say. He was earnest enough, though I'd heard it was bad for a young arm to throw a curve ball. You could blow out an elbow, a shoulder, or something they said. Still, he had me in a spell. "Was it tough being an Indian pitching in the pros?" Maybe we were both strangers here.

"Nah, they never gave me grief about that shit. I was a half-breed anyway. My dad was Mexican. My mom raised us kids in the Navajo tradition after he left us. I just didn't have enough heat to get to the Bigs. That's why I packed it in at thirty-two, too old for ballet, I guess. What's your name, son?"

"Colin."

"What kinda name is that?

"Scottish. It's short for Nicolas."

"I thought you said you were from England."

"I was born in England, but my dad was Scottish. My mum's from County Mayo in western Ireland. I hated my name when we first got here. Nobody could pronounce it right. I asked her if we could change it to something more fitting for America."

"Like what?"

"Cisco."

"Cisco? Like the Cisco Kid?"

"Yeah him, and because Cisco Andrade's my favorite boxer on TV. He's a Mexican. That guy has guts."

"Kid, I don't know nothin' about boxing or Cisco Andrade. Look, here's how you grip the ball if you want to throw the pitch. You curl your first finger under and make it a knuckle. You put that knuckle over these two narrow seams and hold your middle finger away on the ball like this. That finger helps you control the pitch. You'll see."

His face tense now, he made a point like professors I'd know years later. "You bring the ball down off your shoulder like this, curl your wrist and snap it. When I got good at it, I threw the ball at a right-handed hitter's shoulder. If I threw the pitch just so, it ended up on the outside corner of the plate at his knees. You can throw *this* curve when you have small hands. Later, when your fingers are longer, you can throw a regular curve ball if you want to. Now, if only I'd had a heater.

———

The next day I got a letter saying I'd been taken by a Little League team, the Kiwanis Braves of Garden Grove. My coaches were Mr. Horton and Mr. Abernathy. "Report for practice as soon as you can after school on Friday, and bring your birth certificate." I waited for Mr. Navarro to come home from the lumber yard. As soon as I saw him pull into the driveway, I raced across the street waving my letter. "Mr. Navarro, I'm on a team. The Braves! Can you believe it? Just like your Boston Braves."

At the first work-out with my Braves, I saw where I stood. Most of the kids were bigger but slower than me. My hitting and fielding fell in the middle of the pack. A couple of our kids could hit the ball a country mile when they hit it, and we all had good leather. Pitching might be a problem. Our guys threw hard, but not often for strikes.

Looking back on it, Mr. Horton and Mr. Abernathy were good men, but they didn't know baseball. They each had a son on the team. I guess they were paying their dues as I would years later as a dad. By the end of the season, they'd paid them. We won the championship with eighteen wins and no losses because we had the best players in the league. Maybe they did know some baseball or at least how to pick their players.

––––––

A couple of sunny evenings later, we were at it again in Ed's yard. He was working me hard. We had to move to a different spot because his wife said we were wearing out the lawn, though I didn't see the worn patches. "I think you're gonna pick up the knuckle curve pretty quick. You already got bite on it. With the fastball and control you got, it could be a dynamite pitch. You can make it break different ways depending on your arm angle. If you bring it straight over the top of your shoulder, it breaks down in the strike zone, kinda like falling off a table. That's a natural pitch for you because that's how you throw your fastball. So, the hitter won't know what's next until it's too late. If you throw from a release point a little lower, a three quarter angle, it breaks sideways, but still drops some. If you go side arm, it breaks flat with no drop at all. But if you throw it like that, the hitters will tune in and figure out what's coming once they've faced you a couple a times."

Nobody knew much about the knuckle curveball in '52 except Ed Navarro and his mentor in the Negro Leagues. The pitch vaulted onto the major league scene in '72 when a young buck from Texas by the name of Burt Hooton threw a no-hitter in his fourth major league start for the Chicago Cubs. He went on to win 151 games for the Cubs and the LA Dodgers. He was runner up to Gaylord Perry for the Cy Young award as the best pitcher in the National League in '78.

––––––

I loved Ed Navarro, but I didn't enjoy his wife. Well, I had no reason to dislike Linda. Maybe I didn't understand her. She was kind enough, pretty, petite, and busty, friendly to me at first when she said to call her Linda. She seemed smarter than Ed or maybe she just had an agenda. Our houses were at the corner of Emerson Avenue and Spruce Street in Garden Grove. You'd call it a blue collar neighborhood. I'd never understood why we had a four-way stop sign at the intersection because traffic was light. It picked up once Linda started wearing short shorts and a skimpy top to work in the yard. She bent over a lot. Maybe we should've called City Hall to have a signal put in. The guys honked, hollered, and whistled. They pulled over to talk with boisterous laughter, lusty now as I think back on it. I couldn't figure out what she was up to, but it wasn't right.

———

Before our first game against the Rotary Club Indians, Mr. Horton said I'd be the starting pitcher, batting ninth. I was shocked. I'd worked out mostly at second base, hitting lead off. I'd thrown just a few innings in practice. I didn't want to pitch the opening game. I guess I got the call because I threw strikes.

The Indians had a brute of a pitcher going against me. At age twelve, Billy Jenkins was six-feet tall and gangly. He threw wicked side arm pitches as if he had a tautly coiled whip for an arm. And he was wild. On top of that, he smirked as if to say, "You better hit me before I hit you." None of the Braves among us was keen to face him.

In each of the first two innings, he hit a batter, the second one on the helmet. Mr. Horton went after the umpire. "Mike, the kid's gonna hurt somebody, hurt somebody real bad. Warn him to knock it off! Tell him you'll throw him out if he keeps this up."

From the bench, I couldn't hear what the umpire had to say, but the Indians' manager hollered back. "Billy's just naturally a little wild. He can't help it. Lighten up everybody!"

I was the first hitter up in the top of the third inning in a scoreless game. My pitches were working, and I hadn't given up a hit or walked a man. From the on-deck circle, I watched Billy warm up. His pitches were all over the place. Two whistled over his catcher's head, plunking the wooden backstop at the base of a meshed screen. I was musing about whether to bunt for a hit, get a walk, or just live to talk about it.

When I stepped into the batter's box, he sneered at me. The first pitch missed low and away for a ball. I stepped out, knowing it was the only hittable pitch I'd see. I should've tried to line it into right field or punch it through the infield. The next one hit me on the left shoulder just under my chin. The pitch was on me so fast I couldn't get out of my stance. I went down hard, groggy, crying out when the pain sank in. After an eternity, Mr. Horton and Mr. Abernathy looked down on me. Ed Navarro was up there too.

I heard the umpire say, "Sir, please go back and sit in the stands with the other fans. We can handle this."

Mr. Horton said, "I'm taking you out of the game, son."

I came back in a feeble voice, trying to find some bravado. "No, please don't. I can still pitch."

Mr. Abernathy said next. "I agree with the kid, Joe. He wasn't hit in the head or his right arm. If he wants to go, let him go."

I knew Billy Jenkins was due up in the bottom of the third inning, and I wanted a crack at him. I didn't last long on the bases when our lead-off hitter grounded into a double play, and I was out at second base. As I sat in the dugout massaging my shoulder and my ego, Ed Navarro sneaked in, motioning me close with his index finger. From the crook in that finger, I thought he wanted to talk knuckle curve ball, but he wanted to talk fastball.

"Son, when Jenkins comes up, whistle a fastball under his chin. Knock him on his ass! Teach that son-of-a-bitch a lesson. Just don't hit him in the head. We call it 'chin music.' I'll explain to the ump that you're just a little wild, and you can't help it. Lighten up everybody!"

So, here he was, Billy Jenkins. I gave him the smirk he'd used, maybe mine a bit exaggerated. He gave me a toothy grin back as if to say, "Aw, shucks. I was just out of control as usual. Don't take it personal."

Not much of a hitter, he swung slow and late. I didn't want to throw at him, but I wanted him to think I might. I threw the first pitch at his left shoulder where he'd hit me. He went flat on his back in the dust. A knuckle curve was belt high on the outside corner for a strike. He dusted off, got up, and gave me a stare, pointing the fat end of his bat at me as if to say "you're coming up later." The next pitch was a knuckle curve too, but from a three quarter arm angle and thrown at his left chest. He was on his back again, and the pitch was a strike.

I thought about what to throw next. A side arm knuckle curve was an obvious choice. My catcher came out to the mound for a briefing. "Nah, just go with a fastball. He's done." Then, with our newly found coolness, we whistled a fastball in tight, just above his knees. Billy jumped back off the plate, called out on strikes. In return, he threw me a stiff middle finger, flipped his bat and helmet in the air, and was ejected. The game was ours, 1-0.

———

We spent the evening in Ed's kitchen. I see and smell it clear now, sixty years later. Exotic scents bowled me over. "Sure smells good in here, Mr. Navarro."

"Call me Ed, son. It's Indian cooking, just fry bread, the three sisters and ginger. I learned to make it at the Albuquerque Indian School."

"The three sisters?"

"Yeah, beans, squash, and maize, corn to you, and lots of ginger. Linda complains about the smell hanging around for days."

The aromatic three sisters soon gave way to the scent of alcohol, acetone, and camphor in a eucalyptus balm he rubbed deep into my left shoulder. "A liniment Josh Williams taught me to whip up. Better than anything you can buy to sooth pain like this. Wow, Billy plunked you good, didn't he? You got a huge knot right here. I didn't know it was this bad."

He worked away for half an hour. My arm was better in minutes. Every now and again, he'd smile and ruffle my hair with his free hand. Maybe his look was what soothed me. "Ya know, son, I really liked how you handled it when Billy came up to hit. I can get hot-headed. I've never thrown at a batter unless one of my guys was hit first. You have to stand up for 'em, ya know. But you really got him and made your point. I guess only his feelings were hurt the way he flipped you off and threw up his gear. It's good you didn't take my advice. He's a bull. He might have charged the mound with his bat."

Then, maybe intoxicated by a compliment, I blundered in a way that's haunted me since, driving away my first mentor in the New World. "Thanks. My arm's better already. Where's Linda tonight? I haven't seen her for a couple of days."

I knew I'd been stupid the moment it slipped out. Ed glanced at the wedding photo of the two of them on the buffet and smiled. "Yeah, you really got that knuckle curve down. I can't believe how quick you picked it up. And with your fast ball, you're gonna be one nasty son-of-a-bitch on the mound when you get older."

I didn't see him again. A few days later, when I rang the bell, Linda answered. "Yeah, he's gone, long gone. He may or not come back. As for you, don't come snoopin' around here no more."

———

Ed was right. I rode his knuckle hook through college on a baseball scholarship. Without it, I don't know if I could've gone at all. The Los Angeles Angels, starting out in '61, offered me a chance to play minor league ball. Signing warm bodies, they penciled me in for a low level spot in St. Cloud, Minnesota. "Just sign on the line, son. Enjoy those bus rides. They love their baseball in that part of the country."

I bailed out then. Players better than me had gone nowhere, and I wanted to go to medical school. My grades were teetering on an edge after too much baseball and fraternal carousing. Harvard and Johns Hopkins weren't on my list; that much was clear. Something needed to be done, and I hunkered down as a student for the first time in my life. I'd find out next year if I'd gotten in, and then decide what to do. Did I have the brains, the guts you need to compete in medical school? If not, I'd jump at a chance to teach high school biology and coach the baseball team.

After I was accepted, Dr. Ellen Hawkins took me under her wing. Scared to death, I'd called her. "Dr. Hawkins, I'm going to Creighton University School of Medicine in Omaha in the fall. I have a job as a chemist this summer at Kraft Foods in Buena Park. Weekends are free, and I have Thursday afternoon off."

"Wonderful! My partner, Angie Dixon, is a Creighton grad, and she's the best. Don't worry. I know it's a fright. You'll be fine. Join us Thursday afternoon in clinic or at the hospital on weekends. You're one of us now. Just call a day ahead so we know you're coming."

In clinic, she took on diabetics, old timers, kids with rashes and fevers, young people stunned by the diagnosis of a sexually transmitted infection, people who were dying, and people who were lying. Her savvy and how she got at the truth stunned me, though I'd seen it as a kid. She was the doctor I longed to be after reading "The Citadel" by A.J. Cronin.

The high point of my apprenticeship, though perhaps not hers, was seeing Ellen deliver a baby at St. Joseph's Hospital in Orange. Deft in the labor and delivery suite, she barked out orders, shrill at times, cursing like a sailor when she needed to. Nothing was going right this morning. She was frightened, in trouble. After the delivery, drenched in sweat, she collapsed in the chair next to me. Tears fell on her scrub suit as she let go a shudder in a breaking voice. "That was touch and go; and I was scared. I hate breech deliveries. Christ, help me. You never know what can go wrong in that room. Still, it never gets old. Just look at proud papa over there. Look at that face!" Then, she slapped my knee as if in comic relief. "That's my reward for putting up with all this damned stress. You'll love being a doctor, Colin, most of the time."

Ellen was a dynamo. Could I be her? Forget it. I'd never come close.

———

A few years later as a third-year medical student, I volunteered once a week to care for Native Americans on a reservation in Winnebago, Nebraska. A professor I revered led the charge. The natives had a forgiving pride, a gentle ferocity, a noble bearing I wouldn't have seen but for Ed Navarro. They didn't expect much, they didn't get much, and it was OK by them or so they said.

In '72, as a medical epidemic officer at the Centers for Disease Control in Atlanta, I headed up a team investigating a massive outbreak of respiratory illness at the Albuquerque Indian School. Influenza virus, type B, turned out to be the cause, and a student had died of staphylococcal pneumonia as a complication by the time we got there.

Ed had been here. From the aromas in the kitchen, you could tell they still taught kids how to make the three sisters and how to use lots of ginger doing it. One of my colleagues asked, "Wow! What's that smell?"

He was surprised when the answer came from me and not from our hosts, "The three sisters and ginger."

"Who are the three sisters, and who's Ginger? And how the hell do you know anything about it?"

"I'll tell you later."

I didn't smell Josh Williams' liniment though. And where was Ed today? I wanted tell him I still walked in his footsteps and to say "thank you." Had he found another kid to mentor? Maybe I thought he'd be here, coming home in a sense, and that's why I'd badgered my supervisor for this assignment. Ed would've needled me. "So, what happened to the funny accent you used to have when you were that kid from Scotland across the street?"

CHAPTER 2

FIRST DAY AND BRAND NEW

On a date I can't quite recall late in June '67, I was brand new as a medical intern at Harborview Medical Center in Seattle. Two weeks out of medical school, I knew a lot, and I didn't know much. Today and tonight, I'd find out which was worse. Harborview was the county hospital, the most brutal for interns in the University of Washington Program. She took on the rawest of the raw, the vilest of the vile, men and women ravaged by abuse, self-abuse, or just plain neglect. You didn't know who might show up or what for. No frills were handed out, and the patients didn't expect any. At seven in the morning, my heart thumped its way across the lobby to take an elevator up to Station 4C. On a day like this, you're solid, not too arrogant, not too humble, but you can't be ignorant. On top of that, you'd better not lose a soul whose time hadn't come.

The resident I was to work with the next twenty-four hours came by to say hello or maybe to size me up. We were on weekend call, and he had to know the troops. The call schedule was brutal. Residents were on every other night; for a year, they never left home in the morning and returned the same evening. Interns had it worse. We were on call five nights out of seven one week and then two out of seven the next. That way, we got every other Sunday off after living at the hospital the week before. The guy who'd thought this one up must have been a sadistic genius on a tight budget. He'd deployed his troops wisely with no regard for their welfare. Maybe he'll come to the ER tonight with a heart attack or a raging infection. Would we read him his last rights with no resentment?

13

You longed for every other Sunday off, but slept through most of it they said. The committees that wrung their hands and fretted over inhumane treatment of medical house officers wouldn't convene for another twenty years when call schedules were much softer; lucky us.

"Hi. I'm Howie Rubin. How're you doing? How many patients did you pick up?" He was a young Groucho Marx, moustache, nose, eyebrows and all.

"Fourteen, and it's quite a group."

"Show me your list."

He sat down next to me and gave the list a studied once over. "Yeah, I know some of them. Charlie Jackson, an IV drug user who has a staphylococcal heart valve infection, endocarditis. He'll soon need surgery on his leaky aortic valve, if the surgeons will touch him. Alice Monroe with bad hypothyroidism; she showed up in myxedema coma, looking like a frog. She was a Medical Grand Rounds case last week. A thyroid guru from Harvard discussed her case. He sure knew his stuff. Mr. Munford, well only God knows what's wrong with him, if anything's wrong. The rest I don't know, but I get the picture. For sure, your hands are full. Call me if you need help."

He turned to leave, thought better of it, and came back. "And dig in for a Saturday night crisis. Drug trips in Seattle go real bad on weekends. I'll see you later. Nice to meet you, and welcome to the program."

The first order of business after talking to Howie was to meet the patients. As I walked the ward with their charts on a caddy, everyone had a bad cough this morning. "It came on in the middle of the night, Doc, all sudden like."

Still, their lungs were clear, and I saw nothing in their throats. The charge nurse must have noticed my chagrin, bless her. Her name was Penny Nichols, a thirty-year veteran of the foxholes. The patients claimed she was a "short change artist."

"It's your first day, and they know it. They're angling for 'syrup of white pine.' I see lots of bad coughs on this day every year. They can go on for weeks."

"Syrup of white pine?"

"Harboview's cough medicine that doesn't do much, but the patients love the two percent alcohol and that smidge of codeine."

———

By one in the afternoon, I hadn't heard a peep from the emergency room about new admissions, odd for a Saturday the ward clerk had said. Still, I kept busy. An elevator was out, and I helped a colleague haul an EKG machine up three flights of stairs to check on a patient with chest pain. Harborview had no shortage of patients, no shortage of drama, and no shortage of medical know-how among the house staff and the faculty. The shortage was money, and budget crunches held us hostage. Never mind the fondness, even the reverence, the house staff had for the hospital and her patients.

Interns drew blood for tests every morning. Forget about the phlebotomists from the laboratory they have in "real hospitals." The night before, you'd stamped up lab slips, checked boxes, and obsessed over which assay you needed. No automated analyzers then. Every test took a tube of blood. You had to decide for a patient with jaundice whether she needed the test that told you her liver cells were dying or the one that said her bile ducts were blocked.

Too many blood-draws left you a ward full of anemic patients. You got hell about it in red ink from the chief resident, right next to notes that asked, "Rectal exam? Pelvic exam?" Or they said, "You're drowning this patient. Back off on the fluids!" Or, "Scut work builds men. You're an 'iron intern.' Don't forget it, and stay proud." We had no women in the medical intern class that year. Most of them went into pediatrics. Maybe a woman or two would have cut the stench in the locker room.

A shimmering film of bureaucracy kept you from procedures or medications you needed. If you wanted a lateral chest x-ray, a side view to get a better look at the right middle lobe in a patient with pneumonia, you had to call the chief of radiology. She got a lot of calls to hear her tell it, and you'd better have a damned good reason for bothering her.

The only drug on the formulary to treat anxiety was phenobarbital and, of course, anxiety was rampant. If you wanted diazepam (Valium), new and expensive, you had to call the chief medical resident and plead your patient's case and maybe your own. You never knew what sort of response you'd get from the chief resident or the chief of radiology. Still, we were all proud to be here, training in one of the premier programs in the country.

All this at times drove us nuts and led to bizarre behavior. Here's a scenario. After 3:30 pm, the microbiology lab didn't set up the blood cultures used to detect sepsis or blood poisoning. You had to do them yourself in the "intern's lab." That involved melting agar and making pour plates to get a colony count. If you were interrupted and agar boiled over or evaporated, you began again from scratch. One afternoon, I took three blood cultures down to the lab. A couple of pages about nothing delayed me on the way, and I got there at 3:31. The lab tech waved his index finger back and forth like the needle on a metronome, pointed to the clock with a grin, clucked his tongue, and shook his head "no." He'd put in his day. The next afternoon I was down there at 3:29 with twelve blood cultures, pointed to the clock, laughed like a hyena, and shook my head "yes." I never answered a page on my way to the lab again. So it went in the foxhole.

I got a call from the ER at four in the afternoon. "I've got one sick pup down here for you, a 19 year-old girl with fever and lower abdominal pain. Her temp is 104, and she has shaking chills on and off. I can't find anything localizing on exam. I suppose she could have pelvic inflammatory disease or some other sexually transmitted infection, but she only admits to a single partner. Her white blood cell count is 18,000, mostly neutrophils. Blood cultures are cooking. The chest and abdominal films are normal. Can you come down and pick her up? We're getting slammed."

Lying on a gurney, she rode next to me in the elevator. Molly McGinnis, my first new patient after they'd put "MD" after my name, had a fever and a sore belly. I held her hand as we talked our way up to the floor. Toxic and disheveled, she gave me an insecure glance. "You sure seem young to be a doctor. Do you know what the hell you're doing?"

"Molly, we're in this together. We'll get it right."

"Yes, *you'd* better get it right," a voice said in a harsh tone. "She's yours from square one. No bullshit excuses."

I went over Molly with a fine-toothed comb, hoping the teeth were fine enough. The objective findings were fever, lower abdominal pain on palpation, but no "rebound tenderness" to indicate peritonitis, and a high white blood cell count. Taken in sum, the data said she had a bacterial infection, but what the hell was it and when would I know?

Years from now, I'd learn as a physician that the tincture of time was a godsend when defeat and loss were near. But as a rookie that night, impatient and petulant, I had no time for time, and I didn't want to wait 'til tomorrow or the next day for a diagnosis. I'd dutifully made out a list of differential diagnoses, all the possibilities likely and remote. My treatment regimen covered them all unless I'd left something out. So when do we get an answer? I'd like to stop some of these damned drugs. She probably doesn't need most of them.

Her pelvic exam was normal except for slight tenderness on movement of her cervix and the faintest whiff of a putrid odor. I should have paid that whiff more heed. Maybe the ER resident was right; pelvic inflammatory disease or a sexually-transmitted infection due to gonorrhea or Chlamydia. "Let's sit tight and wait for the stains and cultures. She's on two antibiotics," the voice still with me recommended.

I was musing on Molly when I got a call from the microbiology lab a few hours later. A tech was reporting in. "I just happened to notice her blood cultures when I opened the incubator, and I was shocked. I've never seen anything like it! The anaerobic bottles are already cloudy after just a few hours. I did a Gram's stain on the fluid, two different organisms! Looks like Gram-positive rods, a Clostridium species, I think, and a Gram-negative organism, Bacteroides, I'd guess. It has to be a high-grade infection to grow up this fast. That's all I know. I'll keep you posted. Any idea why she'd have these bugs?"

"No, but it's an important clue to *something*. I'll let you know."

She was septic with blood poisoning. I knew a lot of microbiology because I wanted to go into infectious diseases after internal medicine. The University of Washington was renowned for it. Back to square one, I went in to see her again in search of a new hypothesis. Most likely, she didn't have a sexually transmitted infection. That sickening putrid odor had wafted its way by now into the hallway. Rigorous chills and stabbing right chest pain abruptly cut short every reluctant breath she took. How quickly it could all go sour.

"It hurts, and I'm afraid to breathe, Doctor. Help me!"

"OK, Molly. I'll give you something for the pain. They're coming to take another chest x-ray. And I'm changing your antibiotics."

How reassuring was that? How reassuring could I be? "Just keep breathing, damn it. I'll get you right yet," I was thinking.

She'd been started in the ER on intravenous ampicillin and kanamycin for pelvic inflammatory disease. Neither antibiotic would work for an infection caused by anaerobes, organisms thriving in the absence of oxygen. I repeated the gynecologic exam, and she had a thick putrid uterine discharge and jumpy tender areas on either side of her cervix. The chest film now showed an infiltrate (cloudiness) in the right upper lobe, and she had fluid in her chest. When I tapped the fluid as she wobbled on the table, it had that foul odor, and the Gram's stain showed the same organisms she had in her blood.

I changed the ampicillin to chloramphenicol. We knew that chloramphenicol caused potentially lethal white blood cell wipe-out in the bone marrow, but in those days, it was the only antibiotic we could rely on to kill anaerobes. Sometimes all you can do is roll the dice and hope they don't come up snake eyes.

She had suppurative endometritis with septic pulmonary emboli, pus inside her uterus where bugs inflamed pelvic veins and shot clots to her lungs. It happened after vaginal delivery now and then. But she'd never been pregnant, had she? *Had she?* Then, it dawned on me.

She'd had an illegal abortion and was septic with blood poisoning. And she might die because of it. In my angry mind, angrier by the second, a stallion trotted out of a stable, dug a front hoof in the sod, and neighed. I mounted the stallion of justice in a zealous quest for the truth. Maybe I'd only mounted the high horse of self-righteousness. Still, someone would pay for this if I had a say in it.

Molly was coughing up bloody clots now. As she lay there quivering, I wondered if I should anti-coagulate her with heparin. You would, of course, if you were treating bland or uninfected clots to the lung, but hers were septic emboli, tiny but lethal pus-filled missiles launched from her pelvis. I worried about leakage from inflamed veins and capillaries and even more bleeding if she had thinned-out blood. We had no guidelines on this one. Years later, tightrope acts like this would be seen as "risks versus benefits" by professors tapping away on computers. Were they here tonight? I paged Howie Rubin to get his take on it, but he didn't answer. He must have been getting slammed. I didn't start the heparin.

She didn't admit to the abortion at first, but I persisted as she cried out between pained breaths and sieges of violent chills. I felt like a self-righteous jackass, but I had to get to the bottom of it.

"OK, OK, you're right! I bet it's important for you to be right, isn't it, doctor? Aren't you always right? Well, damn you, go to hell!"

The terror in her eyes frightened me. She turned away to face the wall. I couldn't tell if she was sobbing or if the rigors had gripped her again. She turned back to me with a vengeance. "Look, we're not married, and we're not ready for a child. Ramon is out of work. I don't even know if I want to marry him. A girlfriend told me about a lady doctor in the International District. She was professional, and the place was clean, like a sterile clinic; you know, the disinfectant smells you expect. She didn't use a coat hanger on me. I felt safe there. Is that OK with you?"

She tried to get out of bed. I kept her in with an arm around her shoulder. For a moment, her head listed alongside my neck. "OK, Molly. Sorry to be so hard on you. You made a tough decision, and I don't envy you." The horse was back in the stable.

"And I'm sorry for swearing at you. I feel terrible, doctor. I'm scared. Do everything you can."

"Yes, everything you can," the voice said. "You better not let a life slip through your fingers tonight."

Microbiology called again. The blood cultures were growing *Clostriduim perfringens* and *Bacteroides fragilis,* nasty bugs that inflamed veins all over the body. I transferred her to the ICU, afraid she'd need a ventilator if her blood oxygen continued to fall. In those days, you didn't have to turn your patient over to the ICU team. I'd never have turned her over that night, no matter what.

At six in the morning, convinced nothing could be done for Molly or anyone else, I crossed the street to the Harborview Residence Hall to catch a few winks. At eight, the ER called again.

'We've got three more down here; a case of pyelonephritis, who's about to go into septic shock, an alcoholic with some kind of meningitis, and another one with abdominal pain where we can't rule out a surgical belly. We have an orderly on this morn,' and he'll bring 'em up to see you on 4C. Good luck, my friend, and God bless us all. Hell and damnation won't be worse, will they?"

He was right, but it didn't matter. I was here from Saturday morning 'til Monday night. Send me anyone you like; I'm an iron intern. Half awake, half asleep, I made my way back to the hospital. Groucho Marx paged to say, "I know you're overwhelmed. So am I. I'll be there as soon as I can. Sorry I couldn't answer your page."

I looked in on Molly. She was sleeping, breathing easier, and her temperature was down; must have been the damned chloramphenicol. I took away a jar full of the blood clots she'd coughed up, not so much for aesthetics, but so I'd know what was new when I next came by.

While I was pouring over the charts on my new patients, the chief of internal medicine at Harborview showed up at the nursing station. We'd met him yesterday at orientation. He was said to be a hard case, a former third baseman at Kansas. I guess he was checking on the troops, though I'd never seen the chief of any department on a Sunday morning. "You need a shave, Jordan," he said, glancing at my name tag.

"I know I do, Dr. King. Sorry, I just didn't have time last night."

I didn't tell him how much I hated to shave. He reached over the ward clerk's counter to pinch my left cheek, rolled it between his thumb and index finger a couple of times, and said, "Poor baby! Overwhelmed are we? I heard the night was slow. Welcome to Harborview. It can be a hell of a lot worse than this."

The night was slow? Was he hoping it would "be a hell of a lot worse than this?" We'd gotten off to a bad start, and we never recovered.

Later that morning, I was angry, stewing away. Was it Harborview or my internship? Was it Dr. King? No, I didn't think so. Nothing had happened I hadn't expected.

Molly McGinnis had my gut in a vice. How do we get so careless about sex that we cause unwanted pregnancy? Don't we know how conception occurs? When it happens, what should we do about it? Should the woman go to a butcher for a botched abortion that might take her life no matter how medicinal the slaughterhouse smells? What's the man's role in it? I brooded away with nothing to offer. I'd been raised a Catholic and gone to a Jesuit college though I wasn't devout. Roe v. Wade wouldn't be written until 1973, six years away. At twenty-five then, what the hell did I know?

I went to look in on Molly again and again. By afternoon, she'd turned the corner. Only a couple of tiny clots were in the jar, and her fever was down. Heartache was gone, hers more than mine or maybe not. She'd had no idea how sick she'd been or how worried I'd been. She smiled at me. I sat next to her on the bed. "Doctor, I feel so much better. Thank you."

"No need to thank me. Thank the Good Lord. Sometimes, I wonder how in hell we all get home at the end of the day." She smiled again, wearing wire-rimmed glasses now.

"Molly, who was the doctor you saw for the abortion?"

She hesitated and moved away. "You're not going to call the police, are you?"

"I'm not sure. But we need to know who she is, and I need to talk to her."

"Her name is Dr. Alice Wong. I have her card in my purse."

After I verified it with the State Board of Medical Examiners, I was surprised that the abortionist was a licensed physician. I'd always thought they were sleazy back alley banditos making a quick buck or untrained zealots on a mission. Maybe Alice Wong was ahead of her time.

Sex education was what we needed. A couple of days later, I spent half an hour at Molly's bedside going over ovulation, fertilization, and menstruation, scrawling crude diagrams and charts on Harborview Medical Center Progress Note paper. She knew nothing about it. "Can I keep these pages, Doctor, kind of like a souvenir?"

I had no idea she was making fun of me. Molly was an artist who wanted a career in advertising. The next day, she was beautiful, resolute and fiery, wearing make-up, her auburn hair down, dazzling me. I wouldn't have recognized her if I hadn't known which room and bed she was in. She'd redone my drawings. They were stunning. She handed them back with a smile. "You won't have to scribble on that hospital paper again. Give these to your next patient like me."

"Molly, I don't want another patient like you, nothing personal."

Looking back on it with thirty years of hind sight, I should have said. "If you ever watch boxing on TV with Ramon, you've probably heard the referee say, 'Gentlemen, protect yourselves at all times.' He's saying, 'Don't be a sucker for low blows or punches after the bell.' It may not seem like it, but any time a woman has sex, she's at risk. You have to know your cycle and 'protect yourself at all times.' The guy isn't thinking. In the heat of the moment, his brains are between his legs."

After Molly was out of the woods, I took a poll of my peers. Half of them said, "That doctor's a butcher. Turn her in! Call the State Board."

The other half said, "We need help. The problem's bigger than we are."

I kept Dr. Wong's address and phone number in a pocket of my white coat for a few days. Then, I called to tell her about Molly. "She had suppurative endometritis with septic pulmonary emboli and nearly died. We're on to you now. You better knock it off." Maybe I should've asked Dr. Third Baseman to call her.

"I do the best I can for my patients and take every precaution Thanks for not turning me in."

"Alice, I didn't say I'm not turning you in. I have the evidence. If it happens again, we will turn you in, and the State will revoke your medical license."

On the morning of Molly's discharge, I walked her down in a wheelchair with a smile. She deserved the royal treatment. Ramon leaned against the right front fender of his car, smoking a cigarette. For some reason, the sight of him incensed me. "Ramon, she nearly died. Did you know that? Where the hell were you? I never saw you visit. For Christ's sake, use condoms from now on, will you? Molly doesn't need any more shit like this, and Harborview doesn't either."

"I've been pretty busy, out looking for work."

"Glad to hear it. But, from now on, use condoms or keep your pecker zipped up. That's all we ask." Molly looked up at me, her mouth agape, as Ramon and I lifted her into the car.

CHAPTER 3

GREETINGS

On one of those Seattle drizzly days where you can walk the streets for hours and barely get wet, I was back at Harborview. After a few months at the University and the VA, I saw straight away that the number of patients on syrup of white pine was way down. The interns had taken charge, gotten tougher to manipulate, all the more able to take on Vietnam or maybe not. But chicanery by colleagues got your goat as you obsessed about the future and worried about your family. I had a daughter, Teresa, coming up on four then and another, Angela, two months old.

By now, we were used to patients scamming us. Manipulation by colleagues was harder to take. You couldn't be philosophical about it. In those days, most interns went directly into the specialty they wanted as a career, internal medicine in my case, but also family practice, pediatrics, general surgery, or obstetrics and gynecology. Those internships were called "categorical." Later on, you could decide if you wanted to subspecialize in cardiology, infectious diseases, neurosurgery, urology, and so on depending on your tolerance of lengthy training.

But the powers called another type of internship "transitional." Here, the trainee wanted radiology, neurology, psychiatry, or dermatology. The certifying boards said a year of internal medicine or a rotating internship was needed before residency. Fair enough. A radiologist, a psychiatrist, a dermatologist, before he leaves the foxhole, wipes the muck off his hands, and locks the door to his sanctuary, ought to know how sick people end up unconscious on the doorstep and what we do after we find them there.

Still, few "transitionals" had their heart in it. How could you if you were called a "transitional," like a slimy creature with a nefarious agenda in a grade B science fiction movie? Getting from point A to point B as quickly as possible was their goal. One guy, Bernie Scherzer, fooled us for weeks before we caught on to him. He had to do a year of internal medicine before his psychiatry residency. He complained a lot about the call schedule and the "scut work," though he did less of it than anyone else. As an iron intern, you couldn't stand a mate who didn't pull his weight. Before heading home after a night on call, he'd say something like this. "I really got killed last night, no winks at all. Let me sign my patients out to you. My neck hurts really bad today. I'm going home a little early."

Then, he'd rotate his head clockwise as if it were no longer attached to his spine, followed by a couple of cycles counter-clockwise. A tall angular fellow, he usually looked at the ceiling and made little eye contact. He was a hypochondriac on maneuvers. You didn't want him in your fox-hole.

Bernie wasn't ready to sign his patients out to the intern on call. You violated an iron intern's badge of honor if you went home with a patient's IV loose, wasting drug into the soft tissue next to a vein. Bernie had done it a number of times, and I hadn't said anything. Still, at Harborview, with all the financial constraints, you couldn't allow it.

Tonight, after Bernie went home, the patient was a man I knew from a previous night. Ole Olsen was an adorable eighty-year-old blue-eyed duffer, your grandfather if you had the luck to be Norwegian. He'd developed complete or third-degree heart block shortly after he came in with pneumonia. A nurse found him down in his room, screaming, trying to pound the floor; he had a heart rate of twenty-four beats a minute. I was called to see him, carried him back to bed for an exam, and paged the cardiology fellow who came up to the floor and said with confidence. "Mr. Olsen, I've seen your EKGs and rhythm strips. You need a permanent electrical pacemaker now. We can take you right away to the cath lab. Your heart could stop beating at any moment."

I knew Ole wouldn't go for the "bum's rush" by a trainee. He hauled his torso up by way of the side rails on his bed, rolled the blue eyes at the cardiology fellow, and said, "Son, if it stops, it stops. Medicine OK, but no, no fucking pacemaker. I don't like electrical or mechanical shit I don't understand."

After a few hours, the heart block was under control on intravenous isoproterenol, a drug keeping his rate and rhythm up to speed, but a stop-gap maneuver. A couple of nights later, a nurse found his IV infiltrated shortly after Scherzer went home. His heart rate had gone south again. After I replaced the IV and his heart rate had recovered, he wanted to talk. "Doctor, maybe I was stubborn the other night about the pacemaker. I can be like that, Agnes, my wife says all the time. I'm tired of IVs coming loose in my arms. I even had one go out in my groin the other night. Tell me more about pacemakers." He was looking right into my soul, the cunning old codger.

"Ole, they're new, and we don't know much about them. Most pacemakers until now have been short-term hospital devices to get a patient through a rough patch. You'd be getting in on the new permanent pacemakers that should last for years. That's all we know."

"I didn't like the guy the other night shoving a pacemaker down my throat. He needs to be brought down a peg or two like an electrician I know. Reduce him to his real dimensions. What would you do if you were me?"

"I'd go for the pacemaker, Ole. The cardiologists aren't patient. Some days, half the patients they see are on death's door. They can be abrupt, just to keep moving."

"You've been kind, doctor."

He opted for the pacemaker. Logic made sense for once. Two problems solved. No need for IV drugs and no more infiltrated IV lines.

Furious the next morning, I went after Scherzer in the office we shared with two other interns. I should have talked to him in private, but I'd been "killed last night with no winks at all," and I didn't mind embarrassing him in front of colleagues. I didn't roll my neck in either direction before saying, "Bernie, that's the fourth or fifth time this month you've left the house with IVs infiltrated. Last night it was Ole Olsen, and he nearly died, again."

Eli Levinthal, my resident, chimed in. "Yeah, what the hell's up with that shit? I've seen it too. Why didn't you intern at St. Peter's Hospital to avoid all the hassle before your psych residency? Nurses take care of IVs there. And they wipe your ass and put your diaper back on if you still need it. Shalom. I'm outta here."

Bernie mumbled looking out the window, "I'm sorry guys. I haven't always been aware of the infiltrated IVs."

"Bernie, do what we all do. Make rounds before you leave the house. Replace the infiltrated IVs, and don't sign the patients out until you're done. And, for Christ's sake, think about what might happen if you fuck up again."

"Maybe Eli's right. I should've interned at St. Peter's. I'm starting to hate this place. I just hope I can make to July."

"We all do, Bernie. By the way, Mr. Olsen's agreed to a pacemaker and signed the consent form. Please call cardiology to arrange it."

————

Later in the morning, a woman in the hospital mail room paged me. "You got a telegram from Washington, DC; looks official. We're seeing a lot of these. Can you come down and sign for it?"

I knew what it was, no escaping the bloodhounds in those days.

"Greetings:

Report to Presidio, Fort Lewis, Washington for pre-induction physical exam on November 5, 1967 at 1400 hours.

Lt. Colonel Richard J. Ackerman (Ret.). United States Army."

He may be retired now, but this hound had been combing the country with a magnifying glass, tracking down doctors in training. They might bolt for Canada before he could sink his teeth into them. It was the worst of times as best I could tell, maybe for a nation, surely for men eligible for the military draft under "selective service," especially doctors in training. A country was angry and divided, violently divided over Vietnam. The infamous "Tet" (Lunar New Year) offensive was just around the corner. The "Chicago Seven" riots at the Democratic National Convention were only months away.

Male physicians who hadn't served in the military were eligible for the draft until age 35, married with children or no children. The medical deferment or 4-F category, if you had a hernia, a heart murmur or were flatfooted didn't apply to doctors.

A male physician in training owed Uncle Sam two years in those days as a general medical officer after internship. Most likely you'd spend one of them in Vietnam. On top of that, medical specialty training programs wouldn't accept you for residency unless you had an "iron-clad" military deferment. The number of deferments was severely limited because the military needed general medical officers and not specialists.

You had choices, but no control. You could do nothing, accept your fate, and go to Vietnam next August after a month of training at Fort Sam Houston, Texas. You could apply for a deferment to complete your residency training and hope that Vietnam had gone away by then, three to six years later depending on the specialty. To do that, you applied for the "Berry Plan" and waited for a dice roll. The results of your application came out in December so that hospitals could fill their residency slots next July with deferred physicians.

My take on it was this: If I'm going to Vietnam, give me an M16 rifle and teach how me to use it. I'd rather die defending my men than be blown away by a mortar shell or a grenade lobbed into a make-shift hospital tent while I made morning rounds."

The third option was the United States Public Health Service, the USPHS, the "yellow berets." The USPHS was responsible for health care on Native America reservations, in prisons, in inner cities, for a network of federal hospitals, the Coast Guard, the Centers for Disease Control (CDC) in Atlanta, and the National Institutes of Health (NIH) in Bethesda, Maryland. The latter two assignments were in preventive medicine and epidemic investigation or in laboratory research respectively rather than patient care. Competition was fierce, and only men at the top of their class qualified. Every house officer in the country was working an angle, depending on his class ranking. It didn't seem fair to me, but nothing was fair then.

I'd applied for the Berry Plan and a deferment through the USPHS as we all had. When I interviewed for a position at the NIH to work on a leukemia virus of mice, the incumbent two-year officer said. "Don't take this job even if you it means you go to Vietnam. I sit here ten hours a day in a damned space suit changing fluids on viral cultures. I have no input into the research. They don't listen to me in lab meetings. I'm a glorified technician, slave labor, a flunky. And I'm a board-certified oncologist."

I guess every option had a down side. They offered me the position, a way to avoid Vietnam, and I refused it. Later on, the Centers for Disease Control called to say they wanted me as an officer in the Epidemic Intelligence Service (EIS), though they couldn't tell me what the assignment was, where I'd be stationed, or how long my deferment would be. The EIS had been started by Dr. Alexander Langmuir in 1951 because of concerns about bioterrorism during the Korean War.

Over the years, the program had become a sophisticated unit investigating communicable diseases like tuberculosis, out-breaks of infection such as plague, anthrax or meningococcal meningitis, vaccines, tuberculosis, rubella, and measles. A number of EIS alumni were prominent faculty members in medical schools or directors of state health departments. With my interest in infectious diseases, it would be perfect. But, because I didn't yet have a commission as an officer in the USPHS, I was still low hanging fruit for the military draft.

————

When you're an intern, all street-smart and naive, a faculty mentor can set you on a course you never let go. The first mentor I recall, bless him, was Dr. Leonard Cobb, a cardiologist at Harborview. He embarrassed my resident Eli Levinthal and me no end one morning. We'd been on call for the night admitting nine patients. Neither of us had gone to bed. Eli was eager to finish attending physician rounds the day Cobb took over. He had patients to dictate and work to do.

"Thank you, Dr. Cobb. We had one other admission from a nursing home at six this morning. He's a straightforward case of congestive heart failure with a left bundle branch block on his EKG. We can present him tomorrow."

"No, tell me about him now. I don't like loose ends when I take over a service."

Dr. Cobb was about to become world renowned though we knew nothing about it. Early in his career, he had an interest in saving lives. Nothing new there, but he wanted to save them on the street, in bars, and in living rooms. Inspired by the work of Dr. Frank Pantridge, an Irish cardiologist who'd invented the portable cardiac defibrillator, Cobb set up an emergency system whereby internal medicine residents rode the ambulance to the scene of likely cardiac arrests. Lives were saved. Later on, he proposed to the chief of the Seattle fire department that firefighters instead of physicians be trained for the task. The program was called "Medic I" then. Now, we call it "9-1-1" and take it for granted.

Our new attending physician walked into the room to see Mr. Angus Riley, a ninety-year-old, newly admitted from the nursing home down the street. The place was a source of constant irritation because it seemed to delight in sending us patients who'd been sick for months at six in the morning, the morning you were on call. I've never forgotten Dr. Cobb's first words to us: "Angus sure has a deep voice, doesn't he? And do you see how sparse his eyebrows are?"

I looked at Eli. He looked at me. We were in trouble. Then, Cobb asked Mr. Riley if he wouldn't mind getting out of bed to kneel on a chair. "Can one of you guys lend me a reflex hammer?"

While Mr. Riley knelt there, Dr. Cobb cinched the hospital gown behind him to cover his backside. Then, he tapped vigorously on his Achilles tendons. The reflexes were brisk, but Mr. Riley's heels took forever to return to position. We'd missed three classic signs of severe hypothyroidism, too busy ranting about the damned nursing home. "Dr. Cardiac Arrest" still knew a thing or two about thyroid function or the lack of it. Imagine that. "Thanks fellas. See ya tomorrow."

Eli whispered in my ear. "Don't bother to ask him for a letter of recommendation. We won't get the job."

———

I drove down to Fort Lewis for the army physical with a colleague, Richard Lyons, a "transitional" going into neurology. He'd never let IVs infiltrate in his patients' arms, legs, or groins to go home early with a stiff neck after a brutal night on call. He'd been an all Big-Ten defensive tackle at the University of Iowa. He asked me. "Why do they put us through this ritual? They won't find anything to keep us out of the draft as doctors. What's with these physical exams?"

"I don't know, but they're probably covering their asses."

"It'll be interesting to see what they make of my heart exam."

"You have a funky murmur or something?"

"No. I have benign ventricular bigeminy."

Bigeminy is a heart rhythm in which every other beat is premature, a premature ventricular contraction or PVC. Instead of a normal heart beat which goes in a regular way like this: "Lub-dub...lub-dub...lub-dub…lub-dub." Bigeminy sounds like this: "Lub-dub lub-dub……lub-dub lub-dub"…… and so on.

Usually bigeminy reflects a metabolic disorder, side effects of a drug, or an irritable focus in the muscle of the left ventricle. Rarely, it is a benign condition in which the heart beat returns to normal after exercise. I'm sure Richard had a normal rhythm anytime he thrashed a quarterback on the football field. No doubt he was hoping the US Army had never heard of benign ventricular bigeminy.

———

When we got to the Presidio, interns from other training programs around the state and some from Oregon were on hand. Neither of us expected a reception put on solely in honor of medical house officers. We were about to find out how the U.S. Army could orchestrate just about anything and make it seem almost palatable or even understandable.

The army physician's bronze tag said "Maj. Andrew Anderson." He was a career officer, probably about sixty and a rough customer. His wavy black hair and pencil-thin moustache reminded me of the swashbuckling film star Errol Flynn, long past his prime by then. Anderson's hair was greased down with Brylcreem, as if he'd heard the commercial jingle, "Bryl-creem, a little dab'll do ya. The gals'll all pursue ya." I'd never used it. Brylcreem made a come back in the early '90s. By then, I hadn't enough hair to put it to use.

The "examining room" was a gymnasium. Lyndon B. Johnson hung on the wall behind us. An annoying horn went off as if the first half of basketball had just ended. On cue, Major Anderson announced in a booming voice to set the tone. "In the army, we do physicals as a community of men, real men spoilin' for a fight, doctors, just like we're standing at a fucking latrine with no pussy in sight. Nobody moves unless I say so. Got that? Do you fucking get it? OK, now, let's get started."

We lined up in our skivvies while Private First Class (PFC) Jeremy Willis took our blood pressures and looked in our throats. Then, Major Anderson announced. "I'm going to check for inguinal hernias now. When I get to the man in front you, drop your shorts and get yourself in order."

That damned feeling I'd had in first grade during a "community" physical exam came on me again. Why the hell did doctors obsess like this over hernias in the groin? Did they get a referral fee from the surgeon if they found one? Today, I was six years old all over again, just off the boat from England. I knew Anderson would have something to say about it. Doctors always did. By now, the question was intensely personal and tedious. "Not circumcised, huh? What's the deal there?"

"I was born in England, Major. They don't circumcise boys there."

"How barbaric and typical of the damned Limeys! That's OK, son. Uncle Sam still needs you. Bring your extra bits of skin along when you show up for duty."

He gave me a hearty slap on the back. He'd accepted me in spite of my un-American "trouble down there."

Next was the cardiac "exam." He listened to a single heartbeat on every man in the row until he got to Richard Lyons, who said. "With all due respect Major Anderson, I think you should listen a little longer." The major gave him a contemptuous look as if Lyons were trying to pull something. He listened to six heart beats this time.

"Get on that mat over there, do ten push-ups and come back when you're done." Richard looked like the scolded family dog as he left with his tail between his legs. When he came back, Anderson listened again. "Just as I thought, back in normal sinus rhythm. Uncle Sam needs you too, son. Now doctors, bend over, grab your ankles, and smile. We're on rectal time."

With PFC Willis holding a box of examining gloves and a plastic-lined waste can, Anderson did a dozen rectal exams inside of three minutes, moving down the assembly line like "Rosie the Riveter." After every third exam, he'd say "bing, bing, and bing" as Willis checked off three more boxes.

"Good luck in 'Nam, boys, saving your country and protecting the world from Communism," he shouted as we left the gymnasium. I took a last look at Lyndon B. Johnson's photo on the wall.

————

I was on call that night when we got back to Harborview. My resident was Lawrence K. Altman. I hadn't met him, but I knew who he was. On a rotation at the University Hospital the previous month, I had a patient with osteomyelitis of the spine. The infection started in the disc space between the second and third lumbar vertebrae. Over a few months, it chewed its way into the vertebral bodies above and below, causing fever and dreadful pain. A radiologist had done a needle aspirate of the disc space to get us a culture. It grew *Salmonella san diego*. When I arrived at the hospital the next morning, Larry Altman had a note in the chart.

"GRATUITOUS EPIDEMIOLOGY CONSULTATION"

The note said that "*S. san diego* is the sixth most common cause of salmonellosis in the United States" and offered a three page tutorial on the organism and its public health significance. Altman had been an Epidemic Intelligence Service Officer at the CDC, spending much of his time in Africa working on measles. He was now a senior resident in internal medicine and next year would be a fellow in medical genetics under some of the most exacting minds at the University of Washington.

After fellowship, he became a medical and science reporter for the *New York Times*, and the rest, as they say, is history. Altman is now the dean of medical newspaper writers around the world, receiving a number of awards and honors. If that weren't enough, he published a unique book called "Who Goes First? The Story of Self-Experimentation in Medicine" about physicians who'd experimented on themselves to answer a critical question about a disease they didn't have.

But, before that, he was my resident for a night at Harborview. We sat down at two in the morning to talk about patients admitted with abdominal pain, unexplained fever, jaundice, and pneumonia. In his soft-spoken way, he took them in stride. After we'd finished, I had a blue print to take back to the foxhole. Then, he said, and I didn't expect it. "I heard you ripped into Bernie Scherzer this morning."

I'd made a scene in the fishbowl? "I didn't want to, Larry, but he needed to be told. The guy's a walking catastrophe. Eli Levinthal attacked him more viciously than I did."

"Fuses are short these days, aren't they? Must be Vietnam. And I heard you went with Richard Lyons to the Presidio to see Uncle Sam? How'd that go?"

"About the way you'd expect."

"What's your status in the draft?"

"I'm accepted by the CDC for the EIS program you were in. But I don't have a commission yet in the USPHS."

"Good for you! It's a great program, the best our government can offer. Let me be sure I have it right. You're accepted in EIS at CDC, but you don't yet have a commission in the USPHS? And you got your "Greetings" notice from the army?"

"Right."

"You've come through the tough part, the EIS and the CDC. The rest is bullshit bureaucracy. I'll call Mike Gregg later in the morning. He's head of the EIS program as you probably know."

When I got back to the office around six to write up the histories and physicals on the new patients, Larry was on the phone. "Mike, Larry Altman in Seattle. I have an intern here at the University of Washington who's been accepted by EIS. He had his 'greetings' exam today. He needs a commission from the USPHS pronto. Here's his name. Thanks Mike, and a good day to you."

The next day, the lady in the mail room paged again. "You got another telegram. I've never seen one like this. You're just a popular guy with the feds, aren't you?"

"Yeah, lucky me. I'll be right down."

"Greetings:

You are now deferred commissioned officer United States Public Health Service, rank assistant surgeon (Lieutenant Commander 04) effective 1 July 1970 with two year deferment. Welcome aboard!

Vice Admiral William H. Stewart.

Surgeon General, United States of America."

Over the next year or so, I'd run into Larry now and then during his genetics fellowship. We never talked about that night or his call to Dr. Gregg. Thirty years later, we met up again at a national conference he was covering. He didn't recall the night or the phone call.

CHAPTER 4

WAR, DRUGS, AND THE 'DORF
1968-1970

I was there alright, but I wasn't a "child of the sixties." You hear that phrase even now in 2012 when someone winks at you about halcyon days. You wonder if "Johnny-come-lately" isn't sprucing up his resume. Sure, I smelled the marijuana wafting all over the compound we lived in as medical house officers. Maybe I was a square, going about his business, doing his best to raise a family, and missing out on "the 60s." Or maybe I'd done enough carousing in high school and college. I'd always had trouble "with the latest." What my peers had thought of as cool, I'd wanted nothing to do with. Maybe I was still that kid across the street from Ed Navarro in need of a mentor.

By the end of internship, I'd seen my fill of young people in the ER on brutal drug trips, usually LSD and who knew what. Howie Rubin had warned me on my first day. Most of them were an affluent pain in the ass. I'd rather take on a down and out heroin addict any day. He'd never blame Vietnam or an up-tight greedy society for his impulse disorders, though he'd likely blame something or someone. Maybe I was a walking anachronism. I never smoked a joint until I was thirty-five in Los Angeles in 1977. Maybe my rebellion was just put off a decade. The divorce that year probably had a say in it.

Vietnam was killing us, though I had a hard time polarizing myself about it. You couldn't stomach the nightly news or read the paper. I didn't favor the conflict, but it made a certain sense. If the US wasn't going to stop the domino effect of communism, who was? Or maybe the domino effect was political bullshit. Did the US need a fresh approach? Let the communists take bits and strips here and there, but be ready with our allies, if we have any, to thrash them when all the chips were on the table?

Shaking John F. Kennedy's hand outside the Los Angeles Coliseum after the Democratic convention in 1960 may have done me in. I loved him and took it hard when he went down in 1963, my first year in medical school. But still, I didn't think the war gave us the right to riot or to damage private or public property. Angry anarchists with an agenda had filled the void. I didn't know what the hell any of this had to do with smoking dope or why we later glorified the era.

My internship ended the way it began. Coming down the stretch, our families had a picnic on a lake north of Seattle. A touch football game started up, shirts versus skins. Beer flowed, a lot of beer. When the shirts had a comfortable lead, A team mate, Bob Clarkson, whispered in my ear. "Let's grab the keg, put it in that boat, and row cross the lake." We crossed the narrow part of the lake and hauled the keg up onto a dock. As our colleagues on the other side jeered and flipped us off, we sat there and drank blissfully for ten minutes.

A gentleman came up behind us. We figured he was the owner of the property, and we were busted. "Hey, guys, what gives? This is private property. Are you stupid or something?"

Bob responded. "Yes, of course, private property. We may be a little drunk, but I can assure you, kind sir, we're not stupid."

We put the keg back in the boat and rowed across the lake. Our colleagues mobbed us when we came ashore, forgiving and thankful to have their beer back.

———

The time was near. We'd already put notes on the board for the new interns: "7-6-5-4-3-2-1. THEN, 365, YOU TURKEYS. Good luck with that!"

A week before the end, I sprinted up a stairwell at the University Hospital to resuscitate a patient. Pain in my right calf pulled me down, a charley horse? After the patient pulled through, the pain was still there, and I pulled up the pants leg. My calf was flaming red, and I had a thick tender "cord" beneath the muscle; deep-vein thrombophlebitis, I knew. I'd been on my feet from Saturday morning to Monday night.

I went to the chief resident who examined my leg. "We're going to admit you. Get a tourniquet and some red-topped blood tubes, a green-top, and a blue-top. I'll draw the blood. Then, go to the interns' lab, and do a complete blood count, a sedimentation rate, electrolytes and creatinine, and a baseline Lee-White clotting time. We're starting you on IV heparin tonight. You're an iron intern, right, at least for a few more days?"

After admitting me, Bob Clarkson did a thorough exam and found nothing new other than a fever of 102 degrees. I was lowered into the Trendelenburg position, on my back with legs elevated, my head at the bottom of the tilted bed. I'd never been able to doze off on my back, and I knew I wouldn't tonight, especially in the hospital. After an hour, I asked the nurse to send Clarkson back. "Bob, I can't sleep like this. Can you write me for a "sleeper?" I spent the night swirling in a vortex, awake on and off with nausea, Trendelenburg nausea, the worst kind there is, believe me. I called the nurse to ask for a waste basket next to my bed. I didn't want to cause any more trouble.

Early in the morning, the rounding team entered the room. Dr. Robert G. Petersdorf, known as the 'Dorf to the house staff, was in charge. He was chairman of the Department of Internal Medicine at the University of Washington and a renowned figure in infectious diseases. He was why I'd come here.

"Sorry to hear about this, Jordan. You'll get a lung scan this afternoon to make sure you didn't have a pulmonary embolus. Let me see your leg. I heard it was pretty nasty." He pulled the covers back and squeezed my calf so hard I nearly went through the ceiling. I didn't make a sound. A couple of hours later, Bob came back. "You OK? The 'Dorf was a little rough, wasn't he? I thought you were going to go for the chandelier. Do you need a sleeper again tonight?"

"Bob, what was that you gave me? I had vertigo and nausea all night. Can you try something else?"

"OK, sure. It was secobarbital (Seconal, a short-acting barbiturate). No one's ever complained before, your Lordship. I'll give you something else if you agree to a spinal tap to make sure you didn't bleed into your brain because of the heparin!"

After the coagulation tests stabilized, the team discharged me on warfarin sodium (Coumadin), an oral anti-coagulant, literally rat poison, developed by the Wisconsin Alumni Research Foundation. I was ready

37

now for the last five days of internship. I took warfarin for six months, making sure not to slit my throat shaving.

———

You learn early on that a patient in your keep for a night is a sacred trust. You're there to gut it out even when the ice you're both skating on is thin and growing thinner. The darkest moments of my internship came on its last night and the next morning. Peggy Connor was twenty with her bountiful black hair in ringlets and her pale brow beaded in sweat. Lupus and kidney failure had her bloated and gasping for air. Fluid filled her lungs, and her kidneys were gone. She'd been in chronic renal failure for months, but her kidneys had shut down abruptly within the week. She likely had acute renal failure added to chronic, maybe from impaired blood flow. Did we have the time or the means to turn it around?

She didn't respond to potent intravenous diuretics. Bob Clarkson had put a large bore line into the subclavian vein under her right clavicle before he left in haste for his residency in New York. Her only hope now was phlebotomy, judicious blood-letting, then replacement of whole blood with packed red blood cells free of plasma, electrolytes, or extra fluid. I called the blood bank to say we were in for an "all nighter." They got right on it, probably tired of my cheerleading. Every half hour, I took five hundred milliliters (a unit) of whole blood from her left arm and infused half-a-unit of packed red cells into the subclavian line. After six hours, she was breathing easy. By eight in the morning, she was back to baseline, for better or worse. Neither of us had said a word, though she smiled at me when I kissed her dry forehead and left for rounds.

The trouble started around ten when the kidney disease fellow confronted me at the nurses' station. "I'm Jim Kenney from renal. What the hell did you do to Peggy Connor?"

"What the hell did I do to her? She's in her room breathing, isn't she?"

"Yes, but she's not supposed to be in her room breathing. The committee turned her down for dialysis last week because of lupus. As you may not have heard, it's 1968, and we can't take on people with systemic diseases like lupus or diabetes. We can only dialyze patients with pure kidney disease."

I was plenty steamed now and not inclined to be civil. "I know that, but nothing in her chart says anything about a committee decision. What the hell else was I supposed to do? She was drowning."

"Well then, let's take a careful look at the record together, shall we? I dictated that note last week, and I remember it well, painful as it was." After a few seconds, he slumped in his chair. Incredulous, he cried out. "Ah, shit! You're right, the note's not here. I don't know what the hell happened to it. You did what you had to. Maybe you were even a hero. I'm sorry."

"Humor me, Jim. I hardly met her parents last night, and you know them well. Can you explain what happened?"

"Oh, shit! I've already been through this with them a hundred times. OK, OK, I guess I owe you."

A hundred times maybe, but he'd never gotten to the nitty-gritty. Yes, he'd sent a note into the stratosphere, washing his hands of the matter, but what had he told her parents? You don't do the patient or the family a favor when you ignore the muck.

"Yeah, but come clean and say in plain fucking English not to bring her to the ER again. Tell them she needs to die at home with family close, and make sure they get it."

I walked down the hall to say good-bye to Peggy, dreading it. I couldn't wake her. What did I want to say anyway, and why should I wake her to say it? Likely, she'd think me an interloper if she recognized me at all. I left her room and walked to the house staff apartments in the drizzle. I could only think of that damned note on the wall: "365 days, you turkeys. Good luck with that." Internship was done. And so was I.

———

The first year of residency started July 1, 1968. After a couple of months on call every other night, I wilted even though I'd gotten through a more demanding internship on fumes. I was thinking like Bernie Scherzer sounded when he signed out patients with infiltrated IVs. Still, my neck didn't rotate, and my eye contact was strong. I wasn't rolling ball bearings in my hand on a witness stand in a court martial.

The residents weren't the only ones feeling it. The times and the schedule took a toll on spouses. On a night I was on duty at the University Hospital, my wife Jean paged at three in the morning. "Janet Deutsch, Alan's wife, has gone nuts. She's all over the compound, ringing doorbells. She's got a wild look, and she's manic. I just had a call from her parents in New York City. She's called them every hour, ranting on the phone. They're frightened. Her hair's all spiked up, and her makeup is smeared like she's been crying. I didn't tell her parents. Can you track Alan down?"

Alan was a rotating intern, ready to go into family practice next year. I knew he was in the house because I'd seen him in the cafeteria. I paged him.

"Alan, where are you? I need to talk to you."

"I'm trying to get some shut-eye in the interns' quarters. What's the problem?"

"I'll be there in a couple of minutes."

I told him what I knew. "Go home. Give me a quick take on your patients. I'll cover them."

Janet Deutsch was admitted in the morning to the psychiatric service at the University Hospital with manic-depressive psychosis, now called a "bipolar disorder." She responded beautifully to treatment and made a full recovery though she'd need medication for the rest of her life.

———

My assignment in the EIS with the CDC wouldn't start until July 1970, and I wasn't enthused about finishing my residency before then. Most of my colleagues had a different view, wanting to finish training as soon as possible. I took a position as a fellow in infectious diseases for the year 1969-70 – a brief respite because I would still need a final year of residency in internal medicine to be whole as far as board examiners were concerned. I hoped I hadn't burned any bridges. They'll take me back in Seattle, won't they? They did. Or maybe He did.

We called him "the Dorf" out of ear shot. I'm hardly up to the task of writing about him now, nearly forty years later, after reading his obituary by Larry Altman in the New York Times in 2006. How do you write about a man who mentored you, molded you, pushed you, rebuked you, and yet you didn't know him? Where does the homage come from? I doubt many did know Bob. He was tough, blunt, arrogant and opinionated, demanding and unforgiving if you screwed up. He was witty, clever, sarcastic, and caring. He showed us by example how to write a medical paper, how you review your own work critically and that of others, and how you lead, cutting through bullshit, taking on only what you have to. He must have had a child inside him you'd love to know if you could get Bob out one-on-one for a beer.

As you may have guessed, he was one of the "Gods" in academic medicine. The University of Washington was a relatively new medical school, founded in 1946. The founders and the original faculty members did everything right from square one, unlike many schools started at that time or later. By 1968, the University ranked at the top among medical schools nationally in research funding from the National Institutes of Health. It was right there with Harvard, Yale, Cornell, and the rest of the Ivy League, an incredible accomplishment for a public institution.

As chairman of the department of internal medicine, the most important department in any medical school, Petersdorf was a big part of why. He recruited the best of the best, even outside his own field of infectious diseases. The department was renowned internationally in kidney disease, cardiology, gastroenterology, endocrinology, rheumatology, human genetics, bone marrow transplantation, infectious diseases, and cancer research.

Shortly after he finished training at Yale, he wrote a classic paper with his mentor, Paul Beeson. The paper dealt with fever of unknown origin or FUO, one of the most ruthless perversions in medicine. The patient has an unexplained fever that rages and simmers for months. The final diagnosis may be a painless tooth abscess, a malignant lymphoma or kidney cancer, an abscess in the liver or next to the bowel, infected heart valves with negative blood cultures, an inflammatory bowel disorder like Crohn's disease or ulcerative colitis with no abdominal complaints, unusual forms of tuberculosis, or some type of collagen- vascular disease like lupus with negative tests for it.

In the paper, Petersdorf popularized the term "Sutton's Law," based on his study of a hundred patients with FUO. The law said that biopsy of organs with abnormal anatomy or function was more likely to yield a diagnosis than endless blood testing, x-rays, and scans, probing blindly for a needle in the haystack. Before then, physicians would repeat blood tests for relatively uncommon infections like brucellosis, looking to hit a home run.

Willie Sutton was a notorious bank robber who'd been caught again and again. After one of his arrests, the police held a press conference.

A reporter asked why he kept robbing banks. Sutton said. "Well, that's where the money is, ain't it?"

———

As residents, we came to know the 'Dorf through the rituals of morning report and weekly "Professor's Rounds." At morning report, residents presented the patients admitted over the last twenty four hours and gave follow-up on previous admissions. I went to my first morning report as a resident on July 1, 1968 not knowing what to expect. Interns didn't go to morning report though we'd all heard boisterous and jocular comments from our residents.

Today, a senior resident wanted Petersdorf's take on a patient he followed in clinic. "Do you mind giving me some advice before we start report?"

"Shoot."

"I have a young married woman with severe bladder spasms and urethral pain after intercourse. It comes on about an hour later. She runs to the toilet, but hardly any urine comes out. It's gotten to the point where she's afraid to make love to her husband. Do you have any thoughts?"

"You're at the right morning report. That's 'the urethral syndrome,' probably due to normal vaginal bacterial flora being shoved up the urethra and into the bladder during sex. You can prevent it by having the woman take a single dose of nitrofurantoin (Furadantin or Macrodantin) right after intercourse. I call it the 'after-diddle mint.'"

Another resident saw an opening. He was trying to get a test done in radiology on a patient the 'Dorf had heard about yesterday, but the department was refusing, wanting instead to do a newer but less established test. Petersdorf detested bureaucracy and obstructionism in medicine.

"Sounds like administrative and biopolitical dyspareunia. I'll call them after report. They need an earful. Give me the patient's record number."

Dyspareunia is the clinical term for pain some women experience during sexual intercourse. Most often, it's due to vaginal dryness after menopause or an infection caused by Chlamydia, trichomonas or one in the urinary tract.

Petersdorf was a maestro at morning report even when he was wrong. One day, a colleague presented a man who'd come in with an enlarged heart, trouble swallowing, and diffuse thickening of his skin with all sorts of raised lesions.

The 'Dorf asked: "How do we pull it all together?"

The resident didn't know.

"Well, it's obviously scleroderma with involvement of the heart, the esophagus, and the skin. Next case!" With a whimsical expression of triumph, he pounded his fist on the table.

Scleroderma is one of the so-called collagen-vascular diseases, syndromes of unknown cause like systemic lupus erythematosus (lupus). A few days later at morning report, Petersdorf asked the resident. "So, what happened to our man with scleroderma?"

"Well, you see Dr. Petersdorf, it turned out he was a closet alcoholic. His skin rash was caused by scabies (mites), his swallowing problem was due to reflux esophagitis (heartburn), and he had an alcoholic cardiomyopathy (a dilated heart with thickened ventricular muscle)."

The resident, who seemed a bit embarrassed for the 'Dorf, was having trouble with the truth. No matter. Petersdorf looked each of us in the eye, cocked his head to the left, stared up at the ceiling, rolled his eyes and said with self-mocking irony. "If you live by the sword, you die by the sword. Let it be a lesson. See you tomorrow. I'll be in better form."

———

Petersdorf's paper on unexplained fever led to referral of patients from all over the world to the University Hospital. Most came in on Sunday to begin their evaluation. On this Sunday, a rotating intern, Joel Billings, was taking on the patients. He was in over his head. Rotating interns did three months of internal medicine, three months of general surgery, two months of pediatrics, two months of OB-GYN, and filled in the other two months with specialties they had an interest in or might have need for – orthopedics, emergency medicine, neurology or others. After internship, they applied for state licensure in family practice. You didn't need a two-year residency to hang up a shingle as a general practitioner in those days. I'd admired them since I was a kid, entranced by

Ellen Hawkins. I'd gone to medical school wanting to be one of them, but the battle between microbes and man seduced me along the way.

Joel called the hospital operator to page the 'Dorf about one of his FUO patients. When I heard him calling, I gave a slashed throat sign to stop the call until I'd had a chance to go over the patient with him. He waved me off, as was his right. He wasn't in my department, and I wasn't his supervisor.

He had a paper on his desk about etiocholanolone, a substance that supposedly caused fever of any stripe, and I knew he was in trouble. Joel, don't call the 'Dorf at home on Sunday about etiocholanolone! He doesn't believe the data, and he thinks these guys are charlatans.

For years, researchers had tried to identify "the" molecule that brought on fever as if there could be only one. Etiocholanolone was the current darling. You couldn't find a scientific journal that didn't have a paper on it as if you were checking out at the supermarket, looking at "pop culture" magazines. Medical research has its prima donnas whose agendas get in their way. The experiments were designed to find out what they suspected all along, and they found it. That might have been the first time I understood "human nature" as it applied to the search for truth in medicine and science, the day I was shaken out of a tree by colleagues too quick and too invested to analyze data objectively.

"Dr. Petersdorf, I'm sorry to bother you on a weekend. Do you mind if I run one of your new patients by you. I have some thoughts on what we need to do."

Billings gave a condensed history. The Dorf said, "Sounds like a tough one. What do you think?"

"Well, that's why I called. I just read the chapter in 'Harrison's Textbook of Internal Medicine' on Unexplained Fever. I think we need etiocholanolone blood tests to sort out the problem, but I don't know where to send the blood.'

"Who wrote that chapter?"

"I didn't notice."

"I did, Billings. Go back and read it again."

———

If you were intent on a career in infectious diseases, laboratory or clinical research, patient care, epidemiology and public health, third world medicine, or a combination, you didn't leave the University of Washington without a séance with the 'Dorf.

During my fellowship in infectious diseases, I became interested in herpes viruses. In those days, the family included herpes simplex viruses (HSV) types I and II which caused oral and genital lesions, respectively; varicella-zoster virus (VZV) which caused chicken pox and shingles; cytomegalovirus (CMV) which caused horrific birth defects and fatal infections in transplant patients and any patient with a weak immune system; and the most recently described member, the Epstein-Barr virus (EBV), which caused infectious mononucleosis and who knew what else. I was hooked. To me, they were the future in infectious diseases.

I went to his office to set up an appointment. His secretary, Diane Carlson, protected the 'Dorf. At times, I think she thought she was the 'Dorf. "Can you tell me what it's about? And who are you again? How much time do you need? He's busy."

A couple of weeks later, he told me to sit down. All I needed now was his blessing. "I've reviewed your file, Jordan. You're going to EIS in about three months. Congratulations. You've been an outstanding resident. What do you want from me?"

"I'd like an EIS assignment in viral diseases, combining laboratory training with public health and epidemiology.

"Stay away from virology. It's all pediatrics and public health, not what you want to do as an internist. Stick with bacterial meningitis or infected heart valves, where you can use your internal medicine skills."

"I've always thought that, Dr. Petersdorf, but it looks like herpes viruses are going to be a problem in adults. The paper last week in the *New England Journal of Medicine* by Gordon Douglas from Baylor impressed me. He found herpes simplex virus in the saliva of people with a history of cold sores even between attacks. The same may be true of genital herpes. So, silent shedders probably infect others, spreading disease around like Typhoid Mary."

He cocked his head to the left, looked up at the ceiling, rolled his eyes, and said. "I saw the paper. Gordon's a solid scientist. But it's a one trick pony. Stay away from virology. You're an internist. We haven't taught you what that means?"

—————

A few years later, he wrote a paper in the *New England Journal of Medicine* saying we needed fewer specialists and more generalists who would later become known as primary care providers. He was right on that one, but then he took on his own field.

"If we keep training all these infectious disease specialists, before long they'll have nothing to do but culture each other."

—————

Now that you know the 'Dorf, I want to tell you about his predecessor, the man who recruited him to Seattle. He was a character too but from another genre. His name was Robert H. Williams, the founding chairman of the department of internal medicine at the University of Washington, and the man who'd groomed the 'Dorf to succeed him. His accent out of the Tennessee hills was a source of considerable amusement when he showed up at as a trainee in endocrinology at Harvard Medical School. Eventually, the Ivy League boys learned that Williams was a genius who'd take endocrinology far beyond anything their rigid minds had ever imagined.

I ran into him in the elevator the morning I showed up for my first rotation as an intern at the University Hospital. I thought he was a patient on his way to clinic. He was tall and gangly, about seventy, dressed casually. I wore a name tag saying "Intern, Internal Medicine." After giving me the fondest and most reassuring smile I've ever gotten from a stranger, he said in his drawl. "Hello son. I'm Bob Williams. You're one of the new interns, I see. Welcome aboard and good luck this year. Have courage, work hard, and stay true. What do you want to do in your career?"

I didn't make the connection. He didn't say he was Robert H. Williams, MD, who'd written the classic text book in endocrinology. I fumbled my way through. "I'm leaning toward infectious diseases, sir."

He got off the elevator on the fourth floor. I was going to five. He held the door open a moment to say with a wink. "You'll be OK here in infectious diseases, son. As good a field as there is, lots a stuff happening, never stands still."

—————

When I'd run into him from time to time, he was inclined to talk. With an agenda, he'd button hole a group of interns and pull us into his office. Today, he wanted to tell a story about the 'Dorf and how he'd he recruited him from Hopkins to be chief of internal medicine at Harborview. Williams wanted to groom the 'Dorf to succeed him as chairman of the department at the University. Search committees didn't exist in those days, or if they did, Williams had convinced the Dean to let him handle it. If you'd built from scratch perhaps finest department of internal medicine in the world, would you want a committee choosing your successor?

"It was like pullin' teeth. Bob was stubborn. He kept changin' the rules. He was a pain in the ass. I thought he was just a Yankee jackass, but a damned promisin' jackass with a hell of a pedigree. He kept callin' about the money he'd need to develop the department at Harborview. To be honest, I had no idea how I'd come up with it. One day, he called with a laundry list of concerns. After I'd had enough, I said, 'Look Bob, just come on up. We'll take good care a ya. and I hung up on him.' It was a shock, I'm sure. I'd rolled the dice. He didn't call again, but he sent me a telegram acceptin' the position a few days later. He was here at Harborview on July 1, 1960. And now, ya know, he's a hell of a chairman at the University, better than I was."

Maybe the day we'd met in the elevator had done it. He'd see me in the hall, give me a smile, and motion me in to "come set a spell." One day, he had a mind to talk about how he'd nearly died in the coronary care unit at the University Hospital, one of the first CCUs in the country, put in while he was chairman. He didn't know he'd be one of the first patients. He had a number of cardiac arrests. Despite the morbid subject, he grinned when he said, "Yeah, I'd be layin' there in that damned CCU bed. The lights would flicker, go out, and come on. Sometimes, I didn't know if they were comin' on no more. The dark had me, and I'd go limp as a noodle, but I when I woke up ole Frank was there a pumpin' on ma chest. I was always happy to see Frank. He was a good man, a blessing."

Ole Frank was young Frank Parker, a resident when he took care of Williams. By the time I got to Seattle, he was in charge of the internal medicine residency program for the 'Dorf. And yes, he was a good man who kept us all in check.

A few years later, Williams wrote essays on death and dying. I don't doubt for a moment that the cagey hillbilly was setting up geriatrics as a bona fide medical specialty. Here, the revered warrior speaks ahead of his day on the elderly, death, suicide and euthanasia. His thoughts were published in *PostGraduate Medicine* in 1973. The journal targets residents in training.

"Some more successful individuals dream of the days after sixty-five when they'll have enough time and money to enjoy a better home, pleasurable leisure activities, and travel. In the course of time, however, a significant number of those in this seemingly select group experience loneliness, physical and mental infirmities, and other difficulties. A large number find life a struggle financially, socially, physically, and otherwise. With aging, their problems become greater than ever.

Elderly persons feel keenly increasing social ostracism, financial problems, and mental and physical incapacities. For some, impairment of mobility and communication makes them feel that no one genuinely cares for them, that they have reached a stage in life when they are contributing little if anything. They feel they are a burden to friends and relatives and to society. These feelings combine to make them wish for the day when death will come to put an end to it all.

A patient's wish, shared by family, often is shattered by therapies given by physicians whose only consideration is to extend life. In our efforts to prolong every life by the extensive use of drugs, operations, organ transplantation, artificial organs, respirators, hemodialyzers, cross-circulation, and pacemakers, we must consider whether such prolongation leads to happiness or to great physical or mental suffering for the patient and others."

On suicide:

"Many potential suicide victims, aware of societal and religious attitudes, contend with their problems alone until they reach a state of severe depression, anxiety, agitation and frustration. Then, because of distress and exhaustion, they cannot analyze their problems satisfactorily and, in desperation, commit suicide. It is easy for persons who are not experiencing the same agony to advocate calmness and clear thinking. This is like telling someone sitting on a red-hot burner to ignore what he's feeling and his natural defense mechanisms. If all elements of society understood suicide better, potential victims would seek aid sooner and would be treated more effectively. Much progress can be made toward preventing suicide. Information concerning changes in the brain associated with depression, and about means of correcting those changes is accumulating rapidly. Since most people who commit suicide are sick, we should be less castigating and far more active and straightforward in dealing with their specific problems."

On euthanasia:

"In recent surveys, I put the following questions to physicians and non-physicians: With (1) appropriate changes in laws, (2) detailed consideration of the status of the patient and others by his physician and two or more additional hospital personnel, and (3) consent of the patient or an appropriate relative, or both, do you favor in certain carefully selected instances (a) negative euthanasia (planned omission of therapies that probably would prolong life) or (b) positive euthanasia (institution of therapy that it is hoped would hasten death?)

About eighty percent of the physicians and the lay group favored negative euthanasia. About eighteen percent of the physicians and thirty-five percent of the lay group favored positive euthanasia. However, my estimate is that application of negative euthanasia is too little, too late, or non-existent in more than ninety-nine percent of the instances where it should be applied. Positive euthanasia appears to be applied very rarely and probably should not be applied until public attitudes and the laws have been changed.

The excessive use of all drugs, mechanical devices, and other measures is more appropriately designated 'procrastination' with regard to death than prolongation of life. Furthermore, this procrastination not infrequently takes place against the wishes of the patient and his family. The situation has prompted the growing acceptance of preparation of a 'living will' in an attempt to avoid unreasonable prolongation of life. The time and money devoted to delaying death pointlessly would be better spent helping the elderly to enjoy life while they still can."

Williams died on November 4, 1979 on his way to see a patient he loved. We miss him now, yet he's still here. He was in his seventies, going on thirty in his heart.

———

Mornings were crisp in Atlanta as I took a road to the bastion of public health and epidemiology in America, maybe the world. I had a bounce in my step heading for the Centers for Disease Control, known then as the National Communicable Disease Center at 1600 Clifton Road N.E. For the next three days, the 18th Annual Conference of the Epidemic Intelligence Service was on. I was here to take it in and to find out what my assignment was for the next two years.

April in Atlanta is special when stunning dogwoods bloom, before sultry sets in. And by now, Vietnam was fading in the rear view mirror. I'd agonized about it, but my future had been random. Now, my family would be safe; yet I'd still be kosher, giving Uncle Sam two years. My best friend in medical school, now a distinguished ophthalmologist in New York City who volunteers to operate in Gaza and Central America, had been sent there for a year as a general medical officer. After a few months on duty, he developed a bleeding duodenal ulcer and was airlifted to Clark Air Base in the Philippines. They stopped the bleeding, transfused him up, and sent him back to the Can Tho River Delta. I doubt they'd have done that to any officer in the army except a physician conscripted by the draft. A week after he returned to the States, his replacement was killed by sniper fire as he tried to cross the river to tend to Vietnamese families, a crossing my friend had made every week for a year.

I pondered my future as I walked by Emory University Hospital at 1364 Clifton Road, taking everything in. Public health and epidemiology were fascinating, and I wanted to learn as much as I could. But it was virtually impossible to find a faculty position where you could combine those skills with patient care and laboratory research. Most epidemiologists or public health officials did neither even though they were physicians. I would never give up patient care, and I wanted a crack at laboratory research. How naïve I was then.

I'd called too late for a room at the Sheraton Inn across the street from the CDC. I took one at the Clifton Road Guest House, half a mile away at 1115, a charming place run by a couple, a couple of rebels. Bill the husband said, "We love to welcome you CDC boys to our home with all that's going on these days even if some of you are Yankees. Where you from, son?"

"Seattle, Washington."

"Then, you ain't no Yankee, is ya?

"I guess not. Never thought about it."

Nancy said, "Y'all need to know you can't go into a restaurant in Atlanta after seven without a jacket and tie. If you don't have 'em, ask the receptionist to give 'em to y'all from behind the counter. It won't be the best fit, but y'all will be covered."

―――――

The current two year EIS officers, the permanent staff at the CDC ("the lifers"), and EIS alumni attended the conference. In morning sessions, the two year "infectious disease detectives" presented epidemic investigations ranging from meningococcal meningitis outbreaks, adenovirus respiratory disease infections in military barracks, clustered cases of syphilis in inner cities, plague in hippie communes in New Mexico, a number of tularemia outbreaks, and an outbreak of histoplasmosis due to the bulldozing of starling roosts in Mason City, Iowa. The papers were top notch, and the presenters impressive. I'd never seen so many brilliant young people occupying the same space at the same time. The conference was a course on the epidemiology of infection.

The afternoons were set aside for the incoming officers to interview with heads of various departments at the CDC, the directors of state health departments (the states with the strongest epidemiologists could compete to have an officer assigned to them for two years), and career officers from the USPHS Commissioned Corps. We also had a chance to chat with incumbents currently in positions we might be interested in. In other words, an elaborate mating dance was on. At the end of the third afternoon, you got your assignment, a product of the intensity of mutual interest.

After the first day's festivities, a group of us went to Pitty Pat's Porch for a go at southern dining. We all remembered to wear coats and ties. The building had been a funeral parlor. You came in on an upper level, "The Porch," a vast structure above the dining room where waiting diners could sit on elaborate swings and sip mint juleps. It was named after the porch Aunt Pittypat used to entertain guests in "Gone with the Wind." The dining rooms below were filled with American antiques, giving the place an antebellum feel. I half expected Stephen Foster to come out with a banjo and sing "I Dream of Jeannie with the Light Brown Hair." Hand-held fans displayed the menu in honor of the fans at the ends of pews in funeral parlors in antebellum days. Signed photographs of dignitaries and celebrities covered every inch of wall.

Each of us ordered appetizers and entrées. When the appetizers arrived, the feast went communal. We shared the Shrimp Charleston, Southern Georgia Gumbo, Blackeyed Pea Cakes, and Pecan Coated Catfish Fingers. We stuck to the communal plan for Savannah Crab Cakes, Aunt Pittypat's Fried Chicken, Pork Tenderloin with Curried Peanut Sauce, and Rhett's Mixed Grill. No one wanted dessert. After that and one or two too many mint juleps, we were ready for civil war at the Clifton Road Guest House.

———

The next morning I found out that I'd been assigned to the Kansas City Field Station, the clearing house that ran the Ecological Investigations Program. The Program was a consortium of units all over the country. The Kansas City Field Station concerned itself with fungal and viral infections. Other sites in its jurisdiction included the respiratory virus unit in Bethel, Alaska that studied winter viral respiratory disease. The streptococcus and arbovirus (mosquito-borne viruses that cause encephalitis) program was based in Fort Collins, Colorado. The parasitic diseases unit was in San Juan, Puerto Rico, and the hepatitis virus group was housed in Phoenix. The program was my first choice because of a chance to learn how to isolate and propagate viruses.

I spent the last night of the meeting taking in the Annual EIS Skit "Presented by Thirty Obnoxious and Rebellious Officers." And so they were. The program was bipolar. The officers had long hair and were in full beard, more part a hippy commune than presenters at a scientific meeting. In the early going, they lampooned the federal bureaucracy and made fun of "the lifers," who'd been their life lines. The "lifers" grinned through satire that was downright hostile at times. I wondered what they were feeling, and why they weren't squirming. I wanted to scream at the officers: "Yeah, but it wasn't Vietnam, was it?" Then, the thirty obnoxious and rebellious officers repented and went wistful.

Trios and quartets came up to sing Simon and Garfunkel. The first song was "Homeward Bound." I found out later that it referred to officers with horrific assignments in Africa and Bangladesh. Then, we heard "Bridge over Troubled Waters,' sung in homage to the "lifers" who'd nurtured them through rough times. The finale was the "Bookends Theme."

Time it was, and what a time it was,

A time of innocence, a time of confidences.

Long ago it must be. I have a photograph.

Preserve your memories. They're all that's left you.

CHAPTER 5

SAM 'N ELLA ALL OVER AGAIN
1970-1972

On July 1, 1970, we started the course in epidemiology and public health put on by the CDC for new EIS officers. I stayed at the Clifton Road Guest House because I'd come to know the rebels. Atlanta was hot and humid. The downside was that I was apart from my family for a month. Jean and I had two daughters and a son by then. I couldn't wait to join them in Kansas City.

The course was more intense than the heat or the humidity, maybe more so for me than others. I'd never liked biostatistics. In medical school, whenever a professor gave a lecture explaining the difference between "incidence" and "prevalence," my eyes glazed over, and I tuned out, nodding off. Not so with this course; the difference was learning something to pass a test versus knowing the tools of your new trade, temporary though it may be.

We studied events and demographic data that were fed to us as puzzlers. One turned out to be the sinking of the Titanic with its lower death rates among women and children. We got that one pretty quickly. Another was the population in a community in Florida where it became clear eventually that it was a haven for retirees. We did several door to door surveys, soliciting opinions from the public on vaccines and abortion, analyzing the responses in detail and testing different hypotheses. Arguments erupted as some among us tried to spin the data. The opinions didn't hold up for long as we all learned what it took to be objective and the importance of being so.

In those two years, I realized that testing a hypothesis and analyzing data needed the same dose of rigor whether it's public health, epidemiology, basic laboratory research, or clinical trials of medical treatments. In other words, excellence was excellence, and the truth was the truth if that's what you sought. Now, if only you could apply the same principles to your plumber, your car mechanic, or your competitors in research. You expected more from your competitors, but were often disappointed. The "look at me factor" with a rush to fame, money, or vanity got in the way. They say "it's just human nature" as if no one should be expected to curb or ignore their impulses.

———

The Field Station was a couple of blocks east of the intersection at 39th and Rainbow in Kansas City, Kansas, across the street from the University of Kansas Medical Center. For some reason, it was referred to as KU Medical Center. The patients got excellent care, and the faculty and house staff were outstanding. In other words, the Medical Center was a terrific place to receive your care though not high on the prestige meter or in ridiculous magazine rankings because it didn't bring in a lot of NIH dollars for research. It just didn't deserve to be this good. Imagine that.

KU Medical Center was a life-line for the four of us here on two-year duty to maintain our medical skills, much as Emory University Medical Center was for officers in Atlanta. We faithfully attended and presented at conferences, getting to know the faculty and house staff, gradually making ourselves indispensable for the day to day functioning of the medical center. We kept the future in mind, looking forward to the day when we all went home to finish our training.

It wasn't long before my fellow first year officer Ken Powers and I had a crisis call about an outbreak. I took it on September 14. "Hi, I'm Mickey McGloughlin in Sioux City, Iowa. We've got a big problem here, ten cases of Salmonella over the last three days all proven by culture."

He'd done his homework. Now he needed help for his own reasons.

"What species is it?"

"*Salmonella enteritidis* in all of them. I hesitated to call, and I'm sure you guys are busy. But we had the damned Midwest governors' conference here last week, and three of the governors got sick. The Iowa governor is in the hospital whining to the press and threatening to cut funding for our health department. Can you come up and check into it? I already know the source of the problem, a meat-packing plant across the Missouri River in Nebraska. I guess I need to cover my ass in case I'm wrong. I'd appreciate your help covering it."

The "lifers" had drilled the rules into Ken and me at the EIS course in Atlanta, and our local supervisor, Dr. Tom Chin, wanted to make sure we knew them before we set off.

"It's your first outbreak investigation. Remember, don't go on television and don't talk to the press. The local health officials are in charge. Let them take credit for everything you do."

When Ken and I got off the plane in Sioux City, we were surrounded by reporters. One of them was holding up a copy of the Sioux City Journal to show us a headline:

Fed Disease Detectives Here on Salmonella

"So much for rule number one," Ken whispered in my ear.

That afternoon we met with Mickey McGloughlin to get his take on the outbreak. None of us knew the extent of it yet. A portly balding fellow about forty with a thick pony tail down to the middle of his back, he wore rimless glasses and a gaudy green and yellow Hawaiian shirt. His feet were propped on his desk, and he had an agenda.

"That damned meat packing plant, Iowa Beef Packing, Incorporated, I.B.F., Inc. on the other side of the Missouri is the problem. They started out in Iowa, and then fled to Nebraska without changing their name. It didn't set well with the locals."

I don't know about Ken, but my eyes glazed over. McGloughlin had a vendetta against I.B.F, Inc. for some reason. But it seemed unlikely to be the source of the outbreak. We found out later that the company had a sordid history of lawsuits and violent labor strikes, including shootings and bombings. They may even have had mafia connections when they tried to get their beef into New York City.

McGloughlin pulled his feet off the desk and whipped around in his swivel chair to make sure we had it right. "I've been trying to get that cesspool closed down for years. I even met with the governor of Nebraska a while back. He said he'd look into it, but the asshole did nothing. Maybe he's on the take or they have something on him. The company's still in business, and now I have an epidemic to deal with, eighteen new cases yesterday, by the way."

We dug in for an afternoon in the rigorous disciplined way they'd taught us in Atlanta. All the local illnesses were related to one of the restaurants in the Hilton Marina Hotel in South Sioux City, Nebraska though we had no idea then that the outbreak was national in scope; some of those stricken were employees who usually took meals there. At first blush, widespread contamination of the restaurant and its employees explained the outbreak which was now at eighty cases and would reach two-hundred and fifty. Ken and I stayed at the hotel to size up first hand what was going on, though we didn't take meals in house.

We contacted anyone who'd eaten at the restaurant and had a positive stool culture for salmonella. Tracking them down through credit card records was tough because many were by now in Idaho, Indiana, Washington, Ohio, North Carolina, or Colorado. To set up a control group, we contacted people who'd eaten at the restaurant during the outbreak but didn't become ill. We listed in painstaking detail what people ate or didn't eat, and who was ill and who wasn't. The symptoms were typical of salmonella gastroenteritis: hectic fever and chills, severe abdominal cramps and pain, diarrhea, and vomiting.

We sent out a letter to physicians in Iowa and Nebraska asking them not to prescribe antibiotics. Treatment has no affect on the course of the illness and prolongs the shedding of salmonella in the feces, creating carriers, some of whom might be food handlers. Fortunately, no one died among the very young or the very old, the usual victims because the organism tended to get into their bloodstreams.

What became clear was that every diner who was ill had eaten prime rib, roast beef, or ham. Ninety-four percent of patrons who'd eaten those meats were sick. Next, we did rectal swab cultures on all employees. Forty-six percent of the food handlers had positive cultures for salmonella. We assumed that the kitchens were heavily contaminated, but they weren't. None of the hundreds of environmental samples we collected was positive. Nothing suggested that the IBF meat-packing plant in Nebraska had anything to do with the outbreak. A puzzling aspect was that food-handling within the hotel and the restaurants was impeccable. Employees had not contaminated the meats served to patrons.

Every illness was related to the "Cyclone Room," but none had come from a meal in the other restaurant, the "Hawkeye Room." None had occurred among patrons of the buffet that used meats from the kitchen for the Hawkeye Room. The restaurants served over seven hundred patrons a day at the time. So, the source of the outbreak was hiding somewhere in the kitchen that sent meat to the Cyclone Room.

At one in the morning, Ken and I sat on the floor in our hotel room. We had pages of data on the coffee table and all over the carpet. Maybe fatigue gave us special insight or maybe a bottle of cabernet sauvignon did it. We sat there saying over and over. "Prime rib, roast beef, and ham in the Cyclone Room." Suddenly, we both said at the same time looking one another in the eye. "It's the meat slicer for the Cyclone Room!"

We knew what to do. We went downstairs and cultured the slicer blade, the carrier guards, and the scrap catchers beneath. The janitors cleaning up were surprised to see us at that hour. Two days later, we had the answer. The cultures from the slicer were teeming with *Salmonella enteriditis,* and it was nowhere else in the kitchen.

———

Ken and I gave an overview on salmonella infections to the restaurant employees the next morning, not yet knowing the results of the cultures. He emphasized that the vast majority of salonella food borne outbreaks were related to fowl, particularly chicken. "You can go to your local supermarket, culture the innards of chickens, and salmonella will be there thirty percent of the time. You have to make sure you cook chicken thoroughly. Never eat or serve it rarely cooked."

A young busboy named Jimmy Francis came up to see us after the presentation. He was about sixteen. "Can I talk to you doctors?"

"Sure, son, what is it?"

"You were telling us about chicken. A couple of weeks before all this started, I sliced some chicken on the machine in the kitchen next to the Cyclone Room. The chicken was kinda pink inside. Do you think that had something to do with it? I was one of the first employees who got sick. I brought the chicken in from a fast food place. I'm real sorry if I caused the problem."

The only precedent we could find for an outbreak like this was in Aberdeen, Scotland in 1964. Over 500 cases of typhoid fever due to *Salmonella typhi* were traced to imported corned beef sold in a supermarket. A meat slicer had disseminated the infection.

Meat slicers are hard to clean adequately and, once contaminated, remain so for prolonged periods. Generally, the blade is not removed during cleanings with disinfectant because of the hazard to personnel. A technician from the manufacturer comes out once a year to remove the blade for a thorough cleaning, obviously not often enough.

By now the damage had been done. The Hilton Marina Hotel and Restaurants, sabotaged by a reputation for filthy food handling, none of it true, went under.

On the day Ken and I packed up in our room, the local TV news had a story on the outbreak. The chief of the microbiology lab at the University of Iowa in Iowa City had been called in, news to us. He was representing the State Health Department. Maybe Mickey McGloughlin wanted one last crack at Iowa Beef Packing, Inc. or he wasn't happy with our work. When reporters asked the chief how the investigation was going, he said. "It looks to me like it's all down hill from here. I mean…wait a minute…what I meant to say was… the worst is possibly over."

Ken and I looked at one another and smiled. After a week here, we were ready to go home. I didn't know Ken well then. Over the next two years, I'd come to see him as a salt of the earth mid-westerner, an unguarded and candid soul, and a fine athlete with an easy and reassuring smile. He was Jack Armstrong the All American Boy with depth. Today, I was surprised when he asked. "Can you imagine the shit you have to put out there if you're a politician? Do you think this idiot even knows it's the meat slicer?"

"Probably not."

Certainly not. We'd "forgotten" to tell Mickey McGloughlin about the slicer. I made a mental note to call him when we got back to Kansas City. We went down to the lounge for a beer, signed our tab for the week, and headed to the airport.

On the flight home, Ken wanted to talk about his fiancée who was an intensive care unit nurse. They were to be married in two weeks in Chicago, her home town.

"A song runs through my head any time I think of her."

"What's the song?"

"'This Time the Girl is Gonna Stay' by B.J. Thomas.

We submitted our paper describing the outbreak under the title "Salmonellosis among Restaurant Patrons: The Incisive Role of a Meat Slicer" to *The American Journal of Public Health.* It was accepted without revision. Nine months later, the paper still hadn't appeared in the journal. I called to speak to the editor who said. "We must have let it get away from us. Do you have a copy of the acceptance letter you can send back? I can't find that either. Sorry about this. Oh, and send me a copy of the original manuscript again. If everything is in order, we'll fast track it."

———

The beef that two-year officers had with the "lifers" didn't take long to surface. Programs in the CDC bureaucracy had an annual budget to protect. The Ecological Investigations Program in Kansas City with all its branches was no different. The amount of money in the budget was related in part to how many outbreaks had been investigated. Whenever an EIS officer was dispatched to look into an outbreak, an Epidemic Aid Memorandum (an EPI-AID Memo) was sent out from Atlanta. The reason for the temporary duty (TDY) was always the same: "To consult with key personnel."

Bogus calls came in from health officials around the region all the time. You could tell right away which ones had merit, but you had to run them by your supervisor. In December, 1970, I got a call from a health official in Springfield, Missouri.

"We have an epidemic of pneumonia down here. Half the kids in town are sick."

"Oh, really. Has pneumonia been documented by chest film?"

"Not that I know of, but our general practitioners and pediatricians are sure it's pneumonia based on physical exams."

"Has influenza hit town yet? We had our first two proven cases here yesterday."

"I don't know because we send tests for flu to the State Health Department in Columbia. No positive cultures so far."

As opposed to military barracks, nursing homes, or other closed communities, outbreaks of pneumonia are rare in the general population. It sounded bogus to me. I ran it by my supervisor who said what I thought he would. "I think you should go down there right away and check into it."

"But, Tom, they haven't taken a single chest film, and they don't know if they have influenza in the community yet. They have no school absenteeism data. It could just be the normal flu season."

"Yes, but it could be histoplasmosis or something like that."

Maybe he was trying to uphold regional confidence in the Kansas City Field Station. The thought didn't stop me.

"Can't we wait for more data? I'm not sure anything needs to be investigated."

I was thinking about one of the cardinal rules they'd taught us in the EIS course. "Before launching an investigation, make sure there is in fact an outbreak."

"I don't want you to wait for more data. I took the initial call and referred it to you. I've already issued the EPI-AID memo through Atlanta. You're on your way. Put in for your TDY orders."

"Tom, you're ordering me to go?"

"Yes, I am."

I went to Springfield and spent three days talking to health officials, family physicians and pediatricians, reviewing clinic visits and absentee records at school. I even examined some of the kids with "pneumonia" myself even though I wasn't a pediatrician. I didn't agree with the physical exam findings in their charts. No outbreak could be found. None of the chest x-rays, begrudgingly taken, showed pneumonia. School absenteeism was far less than it had been for the Hong Kong flu pandemic of 1968-1969 and about the same as it had been in the last ten non-pandemic years. In other words, nothing was going on, but protocol had been followed and duly noted by those in charge of the Field Station's budget.

I fumed my way back to Kansas City, seething about the damned "lifers." Still, it wasn't Vietnam, was it?

———

Besides a number of epidemic investigations, some bogus and some frightening, we did other good work in those two years. We did a study of influenza vaccine in patients with kidney failure on lifelong dialysis. Vaccination had always been recommended because they were clearly at higher risk of dying during influenza epidemics. But their immune systems were depressed from a toxic metabolic state, and we had no idea if they could respond to the vaccine. In the study we did, their immune system was slightly blunted, but flu shots made sense.

In those two years, my interest in cytomegalovirus (CMV) was kindled. The virus caused horrible birth defects when a woman acquired the infection early in pregnancy. Unlike rubella, where a fever, a rash, or arthritis signaled a problem, the mother had no symptoms to bring her to medical attention. At birth the infants had varying degrees of microcephaly ("pinheadism" or small head circumference), severe mental retardation, deafness, blindness, and an epileptic seizure disorder, a completely unexpected tragedy. About fifteen percent of the babies died, usually from CMV pneumonia within a few days of birth. Yes, I could hear the 'Dorf saying: "You see, that's a pediatric problem."

But recent studies said there was more to it than that. The virus circulated widely in the general population, occasionally causing a form of infectious mononucleosis that we were the first to describe in the United States in 1971 after the original description of the disease in Finland. Once a person acquired the virus, usually with no symptoms, it persisted in their body for life, a state known as "viral latency," typical of infection with all herpes viruses. Most of the time, the latent infection with CMV wasn't important unless the person needed an organ transplant or had an illness requiring immune-suppressing medication. Then, the virus "reactivated" from its dormant state to cause a fatal pneumonia or widespread disease, untreatable with medication until 1984. By 1970, it had become clear that the infection was transmitted by blood transfusion and organ transplantation at an alarming rate, ninety-five percent when a liver transplant was done. So, you see, with all due respect, Dr. Petersdorf, it isn't just a pediatric problem.

We found out something else about CMV; on occasion, it was a sexually transmitted infection or STD. When we gave the paper at a meeting in Chicago in May, 1972, our findings were largely rejected by attendees. I guess everyone wanted to believe CMV was a pediatric problem. To do the study, we took advantage of an arcane law on the books in the state of Kansas. Women who were beauticians, cosmetologists, or masseuses had to have an annual gynecological exam and a blood test for syphilis. The law had no doubt been put in place by well-meaning gentlemen to protect them and their ilk from all sorts of temptations and infestations.

A study from Japan came out in 1970 showing a gradual increase in the frequency of CMV in the vaginal secretions of women through the trimesters of pregnancy, probably due to reactivation of previously dormant virus. We wanted to know if birth control pills had the same affect. They didn't, but we stumbled onto something else.

We divided the women into two groups: those who'd come in for the mandated exams, the "conscripts," and those who'd come in because they were worried about an STD, the "worriers." Among the conscripts, the rate of active vaginal CMV infection was zero. In the worriers, it was thirteen percent. As an indicator of past infection with CMV, the worriers had antibodies against the virus at twice the rate of the conscripts. In addition, about thirty percent of the worriers had a history of gonorrhea, chlamydia, genital warts, or herpes simplex virus, type II, but none of the conscripts did. The cosmetologists, beauticians, and masseuses had been wrongly indicted, convicted, and demonized.

The issue of whether or not CMV was an STD was answered with a resounding "yes" after AIDS was described in 1981. The virus caused retinitis and blindness, colitis, and adrenal failure among AIDS victims, all as a result of sexual transmission among gay men.

———

The last major outbreak we took on was the respiratory disease epidemic at the Albuquerque Indian School. I took the call asking for help from Dr. Miguel Espinoza, a pediatrician and a refugee from Cuba. His wife Esperanza was a pediatrician at the school as well. What gems they would turn out to be. I mailed overnight some viral culture tubes after instructing him how to use them. It sounded like influenza. My second thought was that maybe Ed Navarro would be there.

I wasn't up in the rotation for the next outbreak, and priority should have gone to a first year EIS officer. But I wanted this one. I explained why to Dr. Chin.

"OK. I guess I owe you after that phony pneumonia fiasco in Springfield," he said looking a bit sheepish. "I say go for it. Put your TDY papers in."

————

The school was an enchanting breath of fresh air for grades one through twelve. Students ranged in age from six to forty. Some had scholarships to Ivy League schools or to the prestigious Haskell Institute (now the Haskell Indian Nations University) in Lawrence, Kansas. Others only wanted, after years of alcohol or drug abuse, to get a high school diploma, never mind Harvard, Yale, or Haskell.

The morning we arrived, a seventeen year-old girl with influenza B infection had died of staphylococcal pneumonia as a complication, the first of five students to die. When an influenza virus strikes a community, the cause of bacterial pneumonia changes compared to what you see with no influenza around. Instead of the pneumococcus (*Streptococcus pneumoniae*) causing most hospitalizations, *Staphylococcus aureus* emerges as a major threat for unknown reasons. Physicians need to know this because the staphylococcus isn't susceptible to penicillin or other drugs used to treat the pneumococcus. You have to use an anti-staphylococcal penicillin like methicillin or oxacillin.

As Miguel Espinoza walked us around the clinic, an enchanting aroma wafted out from the kitchen. I couldn't help but comment, "Ah, the three sisters and ginger."

"You know about that, do you?"

Then, I looked through the door of a dictation room to see a physician sobbing in a chair. She looked up at me, smiled warily, and made a pushing gesture with the four fingers of her right hand, her thumb tucked under, as if to say, "I'll be fine in an hour or so. Thanks for coming. We need you. Let's talk later. Just go away for now."

Miguel closed the door. "That's Esperanza. She lost one of her favorite students this morning to staphylococcal pneumonia. The student's name was Anna Wilde. You'll meet Esperanza soon."

Soon was about two hours later when she walked out of the dictation room, ready for the foxhole again. From her look, the devastation hadn't left her.

"I'm sorry about Anna Wilde, Esperanza."

"Thank you. She was our best student this year. She had a scholarship to Haskell, and she wanted a career in science or medicine. Anna could have done it, I'm telling you! Now, she won't be able to do it. Shit. I can't stand it. Where's the justice, the fairness, for Anna?"

She turned away, collected herself, and came back, her brown eyes moist again. "Do you know anything about Haskell, Doctor?"

"I've heard of it."

"It's the best chance our brightest students have to be nurtured by their own. The lives these kids lead are a lot like what Miguel and I knew in Cuba. You scratch and claw, and then hide what you believe, keeping your mouth shut to get anywhere. They've had famous athletes at Haskell, like Jim Thorpe. And do you know Billy Mills?"

Was she changing the rules of engagement? I thought so, and I knew why. She took a gamble that I was a sports nut, and I was. She needed to let Anna Wilde go to get ready for the next random injustice. But still, you don't forget the gasps for air, your final glimpse at a face, eyes vivid, and then closed. For Esperanza, Anna was now a gene sequence in her DNA and part of her forever.

"Yes. I know Billy Mills. He won the 10,000 meters in Mexico City coming from behind in 1964, maybe the greatest upset in Olympic history. He's Sioux isn't he? And, Jim Thorpe, well he's a legend."

"Yes, Mills is Sioux. We're on the same page then. I'm glad you guys are here to help us." Yes, the same page. She sat there looking at me like Eva Peron with her hair up in a severe bun. Her eyes weren't severe though.

"Your name, Esperanza, in Spanish, means 'hope'?"

"Yes 'hope,' but hope with expectation. Maybe for once the good and the just will get a reward here on earth and not be forced to wait for heaven."

She looked at me with a certain expectation. I could only smile, and she grinned back at me.

"Call me Espy, like the students do. May I ask you a question about Anna?"

"Sure."

"I know about staphylococcal pneumonia as a complication of influenza. I started her on methicillin. Should I have done something else?" The question was straightforward, but it told me how sound her medicine was. I don't know how many times I've told house staff and private physicians over the years about staphylococcal pneumonia during influenza outbreaks. They never seem to get it and start the patient on penicillin instead of methicillin or oxacillin. And here she was, a pediatrician from Cuba, and she knew. Something was right in Cuba.

"No. Methicillin is the best we have for Staph aureus. You were right. It just didn't work this time, Espy. Maybe it was too late. I'm sorry. I know how empty you feel."

———

Once we knew the cause of the outbreak, we wanted to figure out how many students had been infected, but didn't become ill. No data existed in the medical literature for either influenza A or B. To look into it, we collected blood samples from all four hundred and forty students. We'd come back a month later to take a second sample. By comparing the serum antibody levels (titers) in each of the two samples, we could tell which students had been infected but didn't have symptoms. You could say we'd overstayed our welcome, or we were exploiting the populace. You could also argue that we shouldn't pass up a chance to fill in a piece of a puzzle about a common infection we needed to know more about.

We set up a table in the gym and took blood samples from students in alphabetical order. We were at it for about six hours. In those days, we used devices called "vacutainers" to do mass bleedings. They were messy and would never be used now because of concerns about spreading hepatitis viruses or HIV by using the same needle to draw blood from different people. After you'd taken a sample, a small amount of residual blood remained in the small plastic cup at the base of the needle. Near the end of the session, I was sitting in a chair, pouring a few drops of blood into a waste can lined with plastic when a huge hand pressed on my right shoulder. I turned to look up at a massive young man who must have been six-feet-eight-inches tall. He growled at me in a thunderous almost celestial voice. "That's Navajo blood you're spilling!"

No doubt looking a bit sheepish, I said, "I'm sorry, son, but that's the way we have to do it. I'll try to keep it to a minimum. Enough Navajo blood has been spilled. Thanks for reminding me."

With our precious samples, we headed to the Indian Health Service Clinic to spin the blood down and to siphon off the serum we needed for the antibody tests. The only centrifuge at the clinic was an eight hole countertop antique, functional but mainly of historical interest. We walked over to St. Mary's Hospital to see if we could use a modern centrifuge that could do a hundred samples at a time. Maybe the Good Sisters could help us out. We explained who we were and what we were doing to the laboratory supervisor.

Technically, in a federal investigation of a disease outbreak, we could order him to let us use the centrifuge. He was ready for us, and I thought I heard gears meshing and grinding in his head. "Where did you say the blood samples came from?"

"The Albuquerque Indian School."

"The school is not on State of New Mexico land. It's on Native American land. I'm not saying you can't spin the bloods because they came from the Indian school. I'd never say that. But it's hospital policy not to allow centrifuges to be used on samples of patients who aren't ours."

"No, I'm sure you'd never say that," I said as we turned to leave.

He had me there. I didn't know the rules and regulations. Maybe he heard me say under my breath, "What a cart-wheeling, careening asshole."

We were up all night spinning blood down in that antiquated eight-hole centrifuge at the Indian Clinic, grateful to have it now. After we got back to Kansas City, I wrote a letter to the chief of the medical staff at St. Mary's Hospital who called to apologize for his "overly zealous laboratory supervisor" and to say that we could use the centrifuges when we came back to collect the convalescent blood samples.

———

I pulled the car up next to a squawk box under a massive concrete tower with a fortified turret on top. The tower was at least sixty feet high. A gun barrel, probably the nose of a machine gun, poked its way through an opening of what looked like bullet-proofed glass.

I pressed the button where it said I should, surprised when a woman's voice came on. "Who are you, and why are you here?"

"My name is Colin Jordan. I'm here for a discharge physical exam from the US Public Health Service."

"Let me look. Yes, we have you on the list today, Doctor. You're scheduled to see Dr. Enders, the prison psychiatrist."

Maybe they knew I was nuts. Still, I wanted nothing to do with the psychiatrist at the Leavenworth Federal Penitentiary. I was here for the physical exam I needed for my discharge. Did he know how to do a physical exam after that "transitional" internship required for psychiatrists?

"Park in the lot over to your right and take the front steps up to the large metal doors. They'll open when you come up. The guard will tell you what to do once you're inside."

Among the notables who'd spent time in this pen were George "Bugs" Moran and George "Machine Gun" Kelly, both mobsters, Leonard Peltier, the Native American Movement leader accused of killing two FBI agents, and Gus Hall, the former head of the Communist Party USA. Later on, Michael Vick, the quarterback for the NFL Atlanta Falcons would come in for running an interstate dog fighting ring known as "Bad Newz Kennels." Oh, and Robert Stroud, the "Bird Man of Alcatraz" was here a spell. I walked up the steps. Massive metal doors opened on cue and clanged behind me like thunder. The doors ahead abruptly separated to give me a look at a uniformed officer. "I'll escort you to the clinic, Doctor. Welcome to Leavenworth. We have to go through minimum security to get there."

"This is minimum security," I thought.

Tough looking customers watched as we walked by. Playing cards or checkers, they squinted up at us. What did the guys in maximum security look like?

When I got to the clinic and took a chair in the waiting room, I began to imagine what could go wrong. I had some dental problems. I'd fractured my mandible playing baseball when I was fifteen. I'd slid head-first into a second baseman's knee that was tougher than my jaw. That same summer, I'd had pericarditis, inflammation of the membrane sac around the heart. A virus caused it they said, but no one could name it. I was the center of attention as the interns at St. Joseph's Hospital in Orange stood in line to listen with their stethoscopes to my pericardial friction rub. And then, during my internship, I had a blood clot in my right lower leg as you've heard. What could come back to haunt me? None of this had kept me out of the service.

When he came out to fetch me, Dr. Enders looked about my age, maybe a little older. In the end, he was more concerned about his problems than mine. He'd read the forms I'd filled out, examined me, and said. "You're fine, no issues as far as your discharge goes when I file the paper work. How's your time been in the USPHS?"

"It's been great. We worked on some outbreaks and got a few good studies done. How's it been for you?"

"Well, it's been terrible, I have to say. Not like you guys in EIS or at the NIH where you have a chance to advance your career. I gripe about it all the time. I'm a board-certified general surgeon. They assigned me here as the prison psychiatrist. I've come to know manic psychosis, paranoid delusions, alcohol withdrawal, and drug-seeking behavior. But I'll need months of retraining before I can take out an appendix or repair a duodenal ulcer again. Hell, I don't even know if I can still deal with varicose veins, for Christ's sake. And I still have a year to go."

CHAPTER 6

THE FIGHT DOCTOR
1972-1973

He wasn't on the radar when I came back to Seattle to finish my training. I would come to know him in an odd kind of way thanks to the 'Dorf. He was Dr. Samuel Ginsberg. God bless the man, and may God watch over any patient he ever took care of.

While stationed in Kansas City, I got two calls from the 'Dorf to offer me a job as chief resident at two different hospitals in Seattle. What an honor it was, and you didn't turn down the 'Dorf, and, for sure, you didn't turn him down twice. I was tempted to give in to the ego stroking, but I held fast. I did my best to explain, and he was more reasonable than I had a right to expect. I worried that as chief resident, in a largely unstructured supervisory position, I'd follow the path of least resistance, looking in on infectious diseases cases and not putting my nose to the grindstone in cardiology, gastroenterology, hematology/oncology, or pulmonary medicine where I'd gone rusty. After three years away from internal medicine, I knew the field had passed me by. At KU Medical Center, the residents were talking about "hemi-blocks" on electrocardiograms and how best to use a Swan-Ganz catheter. I had only a vague notion about either of them. And I still had the internal medicine board exam to deal with, by no means a slam dunk, but you had to get by it or your career in academic medicine went nowhere.

In those days, board certification in internal medicine meant that you wore the same elite badge as professors in academic medical centers. Most internists in private practice had failed the exam at least once, and many had never passed it, a capricious barrier put up by arrogant men in ivory towers. Maybe they thought that no one with any real skill should go into private practice and devote themselves solely to patient care, how tedious and unfulfilling.

The exam consisted of a written preliminary phase that fifty percent of the candidates failed. If you got by that one, you were thrilled to face an oral exam that had a similar failure rate. So, for a physician trained in internal medicine, the odds of being certified on the first go round were around twenty-five percent. What was it that was being certified and for whom? It certainly didn't benefit the patients.

The oral exam was a special problem, capricious and random. Candidates flew off to a medical center in a distant city and then had ninety minutes to do a history and physical examination on two inpatients. Many of the patients belonged to professors at the medical center and had unusual diseases or physical findings, which is why they came in to torment the candidates. Other patients were actually in the hospital to be diagnosed or treated. Most of them had more mundane diseases like alcoholic cirrhosis or rheumatoid arthritis. It was the luck of the draw.

After you finished the history and physical, you sat down in an office with the two examiners. To pass the oral, you had to get five points out of a possible ten. But three points had to come from the senior examiner. If you got three points from the junior examiner and two from the senior examiner, you failed the exam. The junior examiners were apprentices, learning how to torpedo candidates, keeping board certification as difficult and elite as possible.

A colleague two years ahead of me was going for his oral exam to Philadelphia General Hospital (PGH). The chief of internal medicine there had failed over eighty percent of his candidates. Generally, most senior examiners failed about fifty percent. I didn't envy my friend on his way to the mine field. We were talking one day about the patients he might see at PGH. I said. "Harold Israel is chief of medicine there. He's an expert on sarcoidosis, and he probably has a stable of patients to bring in for you to examine, one after the other."

Sarcoidosis, called sarcoid for short, is a disease similar to tuberculosis in terms of the inflammation you see under the microscope but no one knows what causes it. Usually involving the lungs, the joints, and occasionally the central nervous system, it strikes women, in particular African-American women.

When my friend arrived to start his oral exam, he was gratified to know that the first patient had sarcoid. The second patient's diagnosis was a piece of cake, straightforward angina from coronary artery disease. He knew that disease backwards and forwards, and he was ready. Bring on the examiners. While he was presenting the physical findings on the first patient, the senior examiner stopped him and asked. "What did you say about the patient's pupils, doctor?"

"They were round and equal, reactive to light and accommodation."

"That will be all doctor. You just missed Argyll Robertson's pupils. You may go now. Have a safe trip home."

Normally, the pupils constrict when exposed to light (reactive to light), usually a small flashlight, or when they have to focus on an object coming closer (accommodation, in this case the tip of the examiner's index finger). The Argyll Robertson pupils, named after the Scottish ophthalmologist who described them in 1869, don't react to light. He called them "prostitute's pupils;" they occur in the late stages of central nervous system syphilis, twenty to fifty years after the original infection. Argyll Robertson must have assumed that any woman with syphilis must have been a prostitute, a ridiculous notion even in those days. He didn't say anything about men with the same pupils.

Every medical student knows about the pupils and uses a mnemonic to keep them straight. "Prostitutes accommodate, but they don't react." After penicillin became available to treat syphilis in the late 1940s, Argyll Robertson's pupils were rare, and no one expected to see them in a real patient.

———

I got a closer look at the oral board exam that fall in Seattle when the University hosted a site. The 'Dorf, wrapped up in it all, asked me to help bring in patients and show candidates around the hospital. Eighty came to take the exam. I was appalled one day to see one of our local senior examiners stop a cardiology fellow in the hall to ask "Jack, on this chest film, where is the 'reversed three sign' I'm supposed to see in coarctation of the aorta?"

Coarctation of the aorta is a rare congenital condition in which a kink develops in the aorta shortly after it leaves the left ventricle of the heart to supply blood to the lower parts of the body. On certain imaging studies, the kink looks like the number three in reverse. So, here, one of our own revered professors was getting ready to torpedo a candidate on a point he didn't understand himself.

Sometimes, patients with the best of intentions torpedoed candidates. At the end of the second day, I went to a patient's room to say she was free to go and to thank her for coming in for the exam. Her name was Sally Weinstein. Her Crohn's Disease had come on three years ago. Crohn's is one of the two major causes of inflammatory bowel disease, the other being ulcerative colitis. Sally's illness showed itself in the classic way which was the reason she was here for the exam. She started out with pain in the right lower part of her abdomen, next to the appendix. Initially, she was thought to have acute appendicitis until a mass was found on physical exam. The mass was caused by inflammation of the cecum, an intestinal sac where the large bowel begins next to the appendix.

Sally said as I went in to say goodbye. "That last doctor was a sharp fellow and an adorable Jewish boy. He kept asking me if I'd had a mass right here where my Crohn's started," she howled, pointing to the site. "He was getting close, but I denied it!"

"Sally, you're supposed to answer questions truthfully and not hide anything."

I walked to the offices used for the exams and asked the proctor if I could speak to the examiners who'd tested the candidate. They were busy with their last victim. About half-an-hour later, the senior examiner opened the door to release a candidate who was flushed about the face and practically in tears.

I explained to both examiners what had happened with Ms. Weinstein. The senior man said, "Yes, I remember the young man. We examined him this morning. He felt the patient was withholding information and stuck to his guns about Crohn's Disease. He passed with flying colors despite the sabotage."

A few months later the American Board of Internal Medicine announced that it was dropping the oral exam in favor of a single written examination. The clinical skills of trainees would be certified now by the internal medicine training program before candidates were allowed to take the new written examination. The reason given was that it was too expensive flying examiners all over the country and too expensive for the candidates as well. No one mentioned, at least not in public, that it was also capricious, arbitrary, and unfair. But still, the news was all good.

———

My first night on call when I got back to Seattle from Kansas City was at the VA Medical Center. I was on the cardiology service doing night duty as the Admitting Officer of the Day or AOD on the Fourth of July. I was in charge of admissions to the internal medicine ward and for clearing out the emergency room after the daytime career doctors, God bless them, went home. About ten at night, I got a page to come down to see a patient. His name was Johnny Gorman, a ninety-four year-old veteran of the Spanish-American War and World War I.

Some patients go after your heart even if they don't mean to. I'd never worried about the seductive females other male physicians fear when they let their guard down to talk about it. But I was a sucker for the elderly, especially old men. Maybe I saw myself in their shoes one day. When I got off the elevator, the nurse was there to greet me and to hand me the chart. "He's a gem, a special man, ninety-four, and a veteran of two wars. What a cutie pie! Be kind as you can be doctor."

"You don't need to say that. I'll tuck him in all cozy like."

"Hi, Mr. Gorman. Why are you here tonight?"

"They're trying to get rid of me. Call me Johnny, son."

Fearing that I had a paranoid schizophrenic on my hands, despite the adulation in the clinic, I asked, waiting to hear about the voices that come on in the middle of the night. "Who's trying to get rid of you?"

"My son and that bitch he's married to."

"Why would they want to do that?"

"I was working down in the shop today, and I wet myself. It came on too fast for me to get upstairs."

"How often is this happening?"

"About once a week."

"So, you don't have enough warning to get to the bathroom?"

"No. I just try to restrict my fluids before I go down there."

"What do you do in the shop?"

"Wood work mainly. I make bird feeders and little chairs or doll cribs for kids in the neighborhood."

I reviewed his medical records. His health and longevity were remarkable. He'd never been hospitalized except for gunshot wounds in World War I. I wondered about his record of military service, but I didn't have access to it.

I went to the waiting area to talk to his son and daughter-in-law. "He doesn't need to be admitted. I realize what's happening is an inconvenience, but it's manageable. I'll give him a condom catheter. If he has an accident, the urine will run into a bag tied to his leg. All you'll need to do is rinse out the bag and have him put the catheter back on each time. I've explained it to him, and he knows how to use it. The worst thing we could do at his age is to bring him into the hospital. Too many nasty bugs hang out here."

I could tell they weren't happy with my "doctoring." They probably thought I was a quack. An hour later, at one in the morning, I got a page. "Is this Dr. Jordan?"

"Yes, who's calling?"

"Jim Nixon, the VA Hospital Director."

VA hospitals had an odd administrative set-up with a director who had a business or legal background, and a chief of staff who was a physician. They were often at logger heads. "What's this I hear about you refusing to admit a Spanish American War vet and the oldest living Congressional Medal of Honor winner in the United States?"

"Mr. Nixon, he doesn't need to come in. He's ninety-four years old. It's a death sentence. I thought I'd worked out a compromise. I gave him a condom catheter. He seemed happy enough with it."

"What's a condom catheter?"

"He wears a condom on his penis, and if he needs to urinate all of a sudden, the urine drains into a plastic bag attached to his leg,"

"How wonderful! I can just imagine how thrilled the family was about that. I'm ordering you to admit Johnny Gorman to our VA Hospital in Seattle."

"Can you do that without the consent of the chief of staff?"

"I've got you there. She's in full agreement. Call her if you want to hear it for yourself."

I was muttering under my breath, half wanting to be heard. "These assholes, long past their prime, if they ever had one, can make me bring him in?"

"Mr. Nixon, it's a bad decision. He'll probably be sent home with a condom catheter anyway. Or he'll be sent to a nursing home to die. They would probably put in a Foley bladder catheter which is sure to get infected and kill him. Let him go home to work in his shop."

"What was that you said? Do you want me to call your revered Dr. Petersdorf and get him to make you do it?"

"Yeah, call him. I'm sure he'd love to hear from you tonight. Let me know what he has to say."

"I'm calling the veteran's son to tell him to bring in Mr. Gorman right now."

"OK. Alright! There's no urgency, Mr. Nixon. He can come in tomorrow. If they bring him in tonight, it means another history and physical by the admitting intern. He'll get no rest."

"I said 'right now,' didn't I?"

I paged the intern taking admissions to fill her in. "Please make sure the nurses get him out of bed two or three times a day and walk him around the ward or even outside. And check to see that the condom catheter is working. Don't put in a Foley unless there's no way around it."

I'd broken my own rule. I hated calls from residents telling me what to do when I was an intern. For the first time, I knew why they'd called - to prevent a bio-political crisis.

Johnny died of hospital-acquired pneumonia three days later. I went up to the ICU to review the records and talk to the intern. We couldn't figure out what had gone wrong. He'd been out for walks while he was on the ward. He'd gotten respiratory nebulizers. The notes didn't say much. They didn't need to. He was ninety-four years old.

I walked away wondering how much time Johnny Gorman had left for his wood work if he'd worn that damned condom catheter; a week, a month, six months, a year?

———

On my second tour of duty at the VA six months later, this time as a ward resident, we had unexpected incidents. A heavy snow storm hit Seattle in December, paralyzing the city with its steep hilly streets. My intern, James Kleck, and I had spent three consecutive days and nights at the hospital because our replacements "couldn't get in" or so they said on the phone. None of the attending physicians "could get in" either. But somehow, the patients "could get in" by bus from Idaho, Montana, eastern Washington, and even one veteran from Alaska.

On the last night of confinement, Jim and I were sitting in the office at one in the morning. He was dictating histories and physicals on our patients, and I was writing in their charts, covering his omissions. He stopped in the middle of a dictation and abruptly toppled the chart rack over, having a fit. Then, he began to throw charts against the wall. After that, it poured out. "I can't take this shit anymore; the call schedule, the scut work, the dictating, and all this fucking responsibility. Jesus Christ, I can't do it anymore. Good night!"

He stormed out of the office, turned left, heading to the sleeping quarters, I assumed. I wanted to go after him, but I had nothing to offer. I'd see him later after he'd calmed down. I picked up the charts and tried to figure out where he'd left off on his dictations by playing them back.

A couple of hours later, I went to the sleeping quarters. Coming down the hall, I heard Jim sobbing in the room we shared. I took off my scrubs for a shower. When I came back to the room, Jim was sitting on the edge of his bed. He looked up at me with a swollen face and red eyes. "Colin, I'm sorry for the meltdown. Being stranded here has been hard to take."

"Don't worry about it, Jim. We've all felt like that at times. Let's try to get some shut-eye. We should be able to go home later in the day if the assholes can figure out how to get in. We'll take our revenge by introducing them to all their new patients, wishing them well, saying thanks for nothing, and waving good-bye."

At five in the morning, I got a page from a psychiatry resident, a Dr. Fell, who said. "We have a patient on the psych ward who was admitted to internal medicine two years ago with pneumococcal pneumonia. He's been getting intramuscular injections of procaine penicillin twice a day ever since. Is that enough? Do you think we can stop it now?"

"Well, there's been a fuck-up here," I was thinking. But hell, I'd only had two hours sleep tonight, and little more than that in any of the other nights Jim and I had been holed up. I said to Dr. Fell, knowing that I'd check into the problem as soon as I woke up. "Treatment of pneumo-coccal pneumonia with procaine penicillin takes ten to fourteen days, depending on the severity. Is there some fucking reason you had to page at five in the morning if it's been going on for two years?"

———

A few days later, we seemed back to normal, though I was leery of Jim. We had another problem, a life or death problem. Two patients with kidney failure came to our service when dialysis was in its infancy. Much of the basic work had been done at the University of Washington by Dr. Belding Scribner and his colleagues.

We had no openings for patients at the VA. Choices were grim and brutal. Some patients were accepted, and others got a death sentence. As the doctor of a patient with a death sentence, you could watch him die explaining to the family blow by blow what to look for next or you could send him to a hospice and wash your hands; hard to say which was worse.

In those days, patients who had a disease limited to the kidneys were ideal candidates for dialysis. Patients with lupus, diabetes, or any disease involving organs other than the kidneys weren't taken. You knew that when you pulled together your proposal for the committee that decided who lived or died. Ministers, priests, rabbis, local business leaders, and physicians made up the committee.

For today's meeting, both patients on the docket were ours. Typically, the intern presented them to the committee, but I went along with Jim today to make sure his summaries were accurate and, I admit, out of curiosity to see how the process worked. Jim didn't seem to mind me coming; in fact, he seemed to welcome it.

The two best measures of kidney function are the serum creatinine (normally less the 1.0) and the blood urea nitrogen or BUN (usually less that 25). In renal failure, the creatinine may get as high as 12.0, and the BUN as high as 240.

The first patient Jim presented was Casey Cavanaugh, a forty-one year old married tax accountant with two children. He had a congenital disorder called polycystic disease that usually causes kidney failure when the patient reaches his or her thirties or early forties. The disease is inherited as an autosomal dominant condition, meaning that fifty percent of the offspring of either gender will develop the disease. His BUN was 84. To make sure he had his family health insurance in order, the nephrologists had instructed Mr. Cavanaugh to have his two sons checked for the disease so that the company couldn't deny coverage. But at ages five and eight they might have been too young for the disorder to be detected in those days.

The second patient was Jimmy Mahoney, a sixty-two year old ne'er-do-well alcoholic who'd been admitted in a state of profound mental confusion with severe congestive heart failure. He was a charmer, and he was three sheets to the wind. No one knew the cause of his kidney disease because he'd refused a biopsy on several occasions. Most likely, severe hypertension was the cause of both his renal failure and his heart failure. His BUN was 226.

After we'd presented Casey and Jimmy, we returned to the ward for an hour before going back to hear the committee's decision. We both knew what the outcome would be and viewed all this as some sort of bureaucratic charade. Mr. Cavanaugh was selected for dialysis, and Mr. Mahoney was turned down.

I wasn't so much that the decision surprised me, and I didn't have a problem with it. I just wanted to know how they'd made it. I asked the chairman, a banker, why they'd turned down Mr. Mahoney. "He came up with a lot of negative attributes on the Minnesota Multiphasic Personality Inventory exam."

I was thinking. "Mr. Banker, sir, you probably wouldn't do too well on the MMPI if your BUN was 226." Mr. Mahoney never knew what hit him. What kind of cover-your-ass crap is this? Why not just say 'he's a ne'er do well homeless alcoholic' who might not show up for his dialysis appointments and forget about giving him an MMPI?"

Instead, realizing that we now had a new frontier, all I could say was, "I see."

After the VA, I did gastroenterology at the University, endocrinology at the USPHS Hospital which was new to the program, a stint on the internal medicine ward at the University, and kidney diseases at Harborview. That rotation may have been the highlight of my year, the day "The Duke" walked onto the ward. I was sitting at the nursing station writing a note when he made his entrance. I said to a colleague on my right, "Here's John Wayne, the Duke."

"Yeah sure" he said.

I had met the Duke in LA about a dozen years ago. I was a college student pledging a fraternity. One of the senior members, also a pre-med student, was his oldest son, Patrick Wayne. One of my assignments as a pledge was to cook breakfast for the Duke and his wife, Pilar. It went badly, but they were gracious about it.

So here he was again, this time in Seattle, where he was making a film called "McQ" with Colleen Dewhurst and Eddie Albert. They'd filmed speed boat chases that morning on Puget Sound. The movie had to do with corruption in the Seattle Police Department though I knew nothing about it or the movie.

The Duke wanted to visit patients at the county hospital while he was here. A patient he saw was Tony Mendoza, admitted after a horrendous motor vehicle accident. Tony was a pathetic sight, hanging from trapezes, his extremities and head covered with bandages. His eyes and his fingers and toes were his only visible body parts.

The Duke said "Tony, this is a tragedy. I'm sorry for what happened to you. Hang in there. You're going to be OK, they tell me."

"Thank you, Mr. Wayne. I love all your movies."

When he came to the nursing station, Wayne wanted to know what had happened to Tony. The chief resident on orthopedics said "It's a long story. You see, he stole a car, and there was a police chase. Tony rolled the car before the police apprehended him."

The Duke walked back toward Tony's room and barked at him from the hallway. "Tony, Tony! I changed my mind. That was really dumb what you did. Now you have to serve the time. Don't do anything stupid like that again! Ya hear me?"

———

I had hematology/oncology and pulmonary medicine still to do, and I'd be on my way to the University Hospital in Los Angeles to take a faculty position. Or so I thought until I got a page from the 'Dorf in late February. "Do you remember the calls I made to offer you two of my chief residency positions when you were in Kansas City?"

"Yes, of course. I was very flattered. You aren't mad at me, are you?"

"I was for a while, but now I'm calling to say that you *will* be a chief resident the rest of your time here."

I was surprised but had no way out, judging from his tone. I wondered if something had happened to one of our current chief residents.

"We're taking over the training program at St. Peter's Hospital downtown. We want to grow our residency, and we need those beds. They have eight rotating interns, a lazy bunch, I hear. The hospital was just put on probation for program deficiencies. You'll be the only University house officer there for the next four months. Whip things into shape and get the lay of the land. Report back to me. You won't have your last two rotations. You'll just have to study heme-onc and pulmonary medicine extra hard while you're at St. Peter's. If you do that, you should be OK for your internal medicine boards. Thanks for agreeing, Jordan."

———

In my medical training, I'd never spent a second in a private hospital, a place where community physicians ran the show, a place not teeming with bright young house officers obsessing over every decision they made or full-time faculty members questioning their every move. I knew it would be different; I just didn't know how different.

This is where Dr. Samuel Ginzberg comes in. The chief of the hospital's medical staff paged me and asked me to come to his office the morning I showed up. His name was Mel Worth, a general surgeon.

"Welcome to St. Peter's. Thanks for coming over. We hope your time here will be well spent."

"Thanks. I'm happy to be here."

"Did Dr. Petersdorf say anything to you about Dr. Ginzberg?"

"No, he didn't."

"Well, he's become a problem for us. Petersdorf said you were the perfect person to deal with him."

"Terrific," I thought. The good old 'Dorf had left something out. I was all ears.

"Do you ever watch the Friday night boxing on TV?"

"Every now and then."

"Dr. Ginzberg is the fight doctor, you know the doctor the referee calls into the ring to look at a cut around a fighter's eye. The fight doctor decides if the match should be stopped."

"Oh yes. I've seen him. Dr. Sam, the announcers call him."

"That's right. He's also the doctor at the Long Acres horse racing track. But we've had concerns about his practice for a few years now. He's seventy and should probably retire. We'd like you to keep an eye on him, go over his orders, his medical prescribing, and so on. I'll back you all the way if you think something needs to be done to limit his privileges to certain kinds of patients or if you think his privileges need to be terminated. It won't be easy though. His patients love him."

Here I was trying to finish my residency in some kind of normal fashion. I didn't need another headache. The credentialing committees that monitored the competence of a hospital's medical staff were only starting to form in 1973. Until they were at full throttle, problems were handled with a sort of informal spy network. I didn't want any part of it, and I didn't like being used. I especially didn't like being misused.

———

Later that morning, I took the elevator up to the sixth floor where I was to meet the eight interns I'd be supervising. When the elevator door opened, I smelled it, the same putrid stench Molly McGinnis had given off after her septic abortion. An anaerobic infection was festering somewhere on this floor, but no one else seemed to know it. The nurses were going their about business. I poked my head into the conference room reserved for our meeting and said to the interns:

"Hi, I'm Colin Jordan from the University. Something's wrong on this floor – an anaerobic infection somewhere. Can a couple of you come with me?"

I turned left out of the conference room, and the stench lessened after I'd walked about thirty feet. I reversed myself and went right with eight interns following me as if I were the Pied Piper. The stench got stronger. We got to the last room on the left, and a middle-aged man with a cast on his right leg from foot to hip was shaking with chills and hyperventilating. "Jesus Christ! Do any of you guys know this patient?"

One of them said, "Yes, he's Mr. Atkins, a juvenile diabetic. He had surgery on his fractured tibia about a week ago. He looked fine yesterday."

I wasn't in a mood to be diplomatic. "He's probably got gas gangrene from an anaerobic infection under the cast and maybe diabetic ketoacidosis from the looks of his breathing. Somebody get a fucking saw and cut the damned cast off. Somebody else call his attending physician. He's going to the ICU. Didn't any of you idiots notice the stench?"

Then, it occurred to me that Mr. Atkins might have heard my tantrum. Not good. No, he was too delirious to hear anything. "And he needs a lumbar puncture to rule out meningitis, damn it!"

Mr. Atkins survived but without his right leg.

―――

A few hours later, one of the interns, Jonathan Lester, came by to see me in my makeshift office.

"You were impressive this morning."

"Yeah, if you like to see the new chief resident have a fit in front of a patient."

"No, I mean it. You come from a program at another level compared to what we have here. I applied for a University internship, but I didn't get in. My last two years of medical school were tough. My wife and I had a child. She had toxemia of pregnancy and nearly died. Then she had a post-partum hemorrhage. It all threw me out of synch. I came to St. Peter's because we wanted to be in Seattle. I'm transferring to the Virginia Mason program next year. I want to go into academic nephrology. The University would be a great place to train."

He did just that and made quite a career for himself. We became fast friends with me as mentor and him a reluctant trainee who was probably smarter than I was. We developed a style of interaction where each of us would quiz the other. Senator Sam Ervin conducted the Watergate hearings on TV. We'd sit in the doctors' lounge a while, eat breakfast, and listen to private physicians hoot and hiss at Ervin.

Then, one of us would turn to the other, asking something like this. "What do you think of when a patient comes in after a grand mal epileptic seizure, and you see 'ash leaf' lesions on his skin?"

"Tuberous sclerosis."

"What is the diagnosis when a patient comes in with tender shrunken ear lobes and the heart murmur of aortic insufficiency?"

"Relapsing polychondritis."

"And what about the guy from North Carolina who suddenly goes blind and has metabolic acidosis, the kind with a widened anion gap?"

"Methyl alcohol poisoning from too much moonshine."

And so it went, every day. *Tempus fugit.*

––––––

I met the fight doctor in the morning. "Son, I'm glad they assigned you to my service. I have an interesting practice. I hope you learn a lot in the short time you're with me. Let me know if there's anything I can do to help you shape up the interns. They don't make 'em the way they did in my day."

He was a charmer, short in stature with speckled hazel eyes, a head of unruly frizzy gray hair, and a seductive smile he used to great effect. No wonder his patients loved and revered him. He was right. I learned a lot. Those were the days when privileges were "grandfathered in." The doctors who'd been around longest ran the show and chose their successors, an era on its last legs, thank God.

After we'd seen his first patient, I was already steamed. The patient had chest pain, typical of angina which indicates coronary artery disease and may presage a myocardial infarction or heart attack. The patient's electrocardiogram, when I looked at it, showed a typical left bundle branch block, a pattern in which the QRS complex is widened. Any third year medical student knew this conduction defect. The EKG had been read by Dr. Ginzberg, who had no formal training in cardiology. He was a general practitioner who'd trained in the 1930s. He had been reading EKGs for the hospital for years and billing for his services. The reading said. "There are bizarre W complexes on this man's EKG. He must be very sick. I don't know what's going on, but in any event, something is terribly wrong with this man's heart."

Why did the cardiologists at St. Peter's Hospital let him get away with it? I'd never heard of W complexes, never mind "bizarre" W complexes. As we were leaving the room, the patient motioned me back. "Son, it's a great privilege for you to work under Dr. Ginzberg. Soak up all you can. I hear he's the best heart man on the West Coast. Be sure to show him the respect he's due."

"No wonder this place is on probation," I was thinking. Then, it got worse. I noticed that the next patient was on a fixed-combination antibiotic called "Pan-Alba," a combination of novobiocin and tetracycline.

Combinations of antibiotics are often used to synergize with one another to create more potent bacterial killing. The synergy only works when both antibiotics are bacteriocidal, meaning that both drugs kill their targets. Other antibiotics are bacteriostatic; they inhibit bacterial growth, but don't kill the organisms. Their effectiveness requires the patient's immune system to finish the job. If you use two bacteriostatic drugs in combination, they may antagonize one another to the point where there is little antibacterial effect at all.

"Pan-Alba" was in this latter category yet the pharmaceutical company Upjohn had promoted it so effectively that it was the most widely pre-scribed antibiotic in the United States, a new level of sleaziness. In other words, many patients treated with the drug got better by themselves with no help from the antibiotic. Dr. Bill Kirby, my mentor in my infectious diseases fellowship, chaired an expert committee that testified before the U.S. Senate in 1970. The committee recommended removal of fixed combination antibiotics from the market, and the Food and Drug Administration promptly did so.

I said to Ginzberg. "Dr. Sam, Pan-Alba was taken off the market by the FDA nearly three years ago."

"I think I heard that somewhere. The pharmacy here keeps a secret stash for me. It's a terrific drug."

"There's another problem. The tetracycline component may be out-dated, and it's very toxic to the liver in that case."

"Oh dear. What do you suggest I use? Chloromycetin?"

"Chloromycetin" was the trade name for chloramphenicol, the toxic drug I was forced to use to treat Molly McGinnis' septic abortion on my first day at Harborview. You said a prayer and crossed your fingers anytime you wrote in the chart for that drug.

"No. It's too toxic, and there's no reason to take the risk here."

"What else can I use?"

"After looking over the chart, I don't see evidence of an infection. I don't think she needs an antibiotic."

From the look on his face, he didn't want my suggestion. Irreconcilable differences were creeping in, and we needed a divorce. After rounds, I went to talk to the pharmacists.

"Of course, we knew that Pan-Alba had been taken off the market," one of them said. "But you don't understand how things work here. The doctors run the show, especially Dr. Sam, who grew up with St. Peter's. Other even more appalling things are going on."

"What would it take to stop it?"

"A directive from the Chief of Staff."

———

A few days later, after another three hours of agonizing rounds, Dr. Sam made me an offer. "I'm the physician for the Long Acres horse race track on Sundays. It pays $250 every week. I can't make it this Sunday. Maybe you could go. If you can, try to figure out how that new defibrillator works. We've had it for about three months, and I don't know how to use the damned thing. Fortunately, none of the suckers at the track has had a heart attack yet."

"I can't do it this Sunday. I'm sorry."

"That's OK. I'm sure I can find someone else."

———

With the passing of days, I saw Dr. Sam as a handful, and for some reason, my handful. And I still had three months to get through. Misadventures continued with poor medical histories, missed findings on physical exam, improper interpretation of laboratory and radiological reports, and poor judgment in the use of drugs. Had his clinical skills deteriorated? Or maybe it wasn't deterioration, but a problem for decades. Were the patients in danger? Yes. Was the hospital vulnerable to malpractice damages? Yes. Did I want to do this any more? No.

I stewed away trying to figure out where to go. I was a resident with no board certification. He was a senior, experienced physician whose patients loved and deified him. Had I no compassion for a life's work now waning? Was it my place to confront Dr. Sam? Not knowing what else to do, I made an appointment with Mel Worth, the chief of staff. I didn't pull any punches, but the ones I threw hurt me.

"I see," he said. "It's worse than I knew. What do you think I should do?"

"That's not for me to say, Mel. I'm a resident. But, if I were you, I'd let him down easy. He's a good man who's done his best, but he's done."

––––––

I was relieved of my duties on Dr. Sam's service and told to concentrate on the interns when the 'dorf called to apologize in his fashion. Except for Jonathan Lester, my new job was no better. In a University Hospital, interns take fierce pride in coming up with a list of potential diagnoses (the differential diagnosis) in a patient, thinking through what tests they need to nail it down, and then how to treat the patient. It didn't work like that at St. Peter's Hospital.

Part of the problem was that every patient had a private physician who called the shots. The interns had no incentive to come up with a differential diagnosis because their suggestions were usually ignored. After a few months, they no longer made the effort. Maybe you couldn't blame them because they were "transitionals" in a grade B science fiction movie.

One evening, just as I was about to go home, an intern by the name of Charlie Maxwell stopped me on the way out. "Can I run a patient by you real quick?"

"Sure go ahead."

He went on to present an elderly woman admitted with fever and pain in the right upper part of her abdomen. "So, what's your differential diagnosis, Charlie?"

"I'm thinking either viral hepatitis or an acute gallbladder."

"Both are possible," I thought, but I didn't like the "either." The list should have been a yard long. We went to see the patient, and I reviewed her chart. Maxwell had failed to notice that she'd had a ruptured appendix complicated by an abscess six months earlier. Her diagnosis was delayed at the time because she had no fever and no pain, a common occurrence among the elderly with intra-abdominal infections. Her right upper quadrant pain and fever on this admission would turn out to be due to several liver abscesses and an inflamed portal vein as a complication of the appendicitis.

———

I was debating whether to accept a faculty position at the University Hospital in Los Angeles. My wife Jean and I made a trip to look at houses. As a hot commodity then, I had job offers at a number of academic health centers around the country. The spot at this University Hospital topped the list. The medical school, though young, had a strong reputation and a professor perfect for mentoring my herpes virus research. Returning to Southern California (Jean and I had both grown up in Orange County just south of Los Angeles) was appealing after ten years away, or so we thought. The reaction from friends in Seattle when we said we might go back was painful with their penchant for outdoor life in the Pacific Northwest. "Hell!" they'd say. "For God's sake, are you gluttons for punishment in that smoggy shit hole? Stay here with us where you belong."

I had an agenda. I wanted to work with Dr. Steven Jackson on herpes viruses. They'd never get it with their values.

Jean and I'd been warned about the cost of housing near the medical center. Most junior faculty recruits had settled in the San Fernando Valley, north of the west side of Los Angeles, a different world, they'd said. We'd been sent to Estelle Lederberg, a real estate agent, by friends in Seattle. After three days searching, we were discouraged. We were thinking of looking elsewhere, even if it meant a longer commute for me. Estelle was in her fifties, had fluffed-up blue hair, and drove a vintage Mercedes Benz with authentic wood paneling at its flanks.

"Honey," Estelle, who shared her name with my beloved grandmother in England, said, "if we can get you into Pacific Palisades, you'd be far better off in a few years. It's the hottest real estate market on the planet. The price of houses doubles every two or three years. The little one I just showed you is darling, and it has your names written all over it. You have a partial view of the Pacific Ocean. You have the handsome young actor playing the next James Bond to your left. Ronald Reagan, the governor, is up the street when he's home. It's the cheapest house on this lane which is perfect for resale and not even on the market yet. I found out about it just yesterday from my spies. What's the problem?"

"It's $65,000, Estelle, meaning $13,000 down." I said. "We have $3000. The house we're renting in Seattle is larger and for sale at $22,000. I have a job there, admittedly at a lower salary, but we could buy that house. We'd be nuts to go for this one."

I'd put it on the table. That's what we had. Seattle was looking good. Maybe our friends were right. Never mind Dr. Steven Jackson.

Estelle sat at the wheel of her Mercedes in front of the house. She was pouring over forms, peering through reading glasses. Jean was in the passenger seat, and I sat in the back. Estelle, seeming to turn over my response a few times in her mind, looked over the glasses at Jean, and said. "I like you kids. You have good heads on your shoulders and a bright future. Here's what we'll do. You put your $3000 down, and I'll give you a $10,000 loan as a second mortgage at zero percent interest. Send me a $100 a month. No one needs to know where the money came from. All I ask is that if you decide to sell the house, I have exclusive rights as realtor to the sale. And, you don't need to sign a thing."

I hadn't said a word about the $40,000 in medical student loans I was on the hook for. I'd tried to minimize them working in private hospitals doing pre-operative histories and physicals for a pittance when I wasn't on call. Jean did hard labor in an office. We didn't come close. Paying up was on the docket as were other atonements.

———

My last day in Seattle, my last day at St. Peter's, and the last day of my residency was the day I became a movie star. Innocently enough, I was heading to the library to photocopy a couple of articles to pimp Jonathan Lester. As I came closer to the hospital lobby, I noticed that the lighting was far more intense than usual. I turned the corner to see James Caan squatting next to a wheelchair talking to Marsha Mason who sat in the chair. A man hollered at me. "Doctor, you're perfect for this scene. If you don't mind, can you go back the way you just came and then walk through again in about thirty seconds? Don't look at Mr. Caan or Ms. Mason. Just go about your business. You looked pretty intense."

After my debut, I asked the fellow for the name of the movie. "Cinderella Liberty," he said. "You'll love it."

———

Armed with my articles, I went upstairs to see Jonathan Lester. He had some articles for me too. He went first. "What's the matter with a guy who comes in with metabolic acidosis, and you see oxalate crystals in his urine?"

"He drank a little more antifreeze than he should have, ethylene glycol poisoning."

I shot back. "You're seeing a woman with scaling skin lesions in her scalp who's complaining of pain in her hands. On x-ray, several digits have what the radiologist calls the 'pencil in cup' arthritic deformity.

"Psoriatic arthritis. I was lucky there that she had the skin disease already. Sometimes the arthritis comes on before the skin lesions. And you can't make the diagnosis. By the way, did you hear that Sam Ginzberg announced his retirement?"

"No, I didn't."

I gave him my hand. "Good bye, Jonathan, and best of luck. Let me know where you want to go for nephrology. You've been great. You'll get a strong letter of support now that I'm going to be a hot shot professor; well, a hot shot assistant professor at least."

CHAPTER 7

THE LOW-LIFE MOTEL
1975-1978

I'd grown up just south and had gone to college here. You'd think I'd know what I was getting into in LA, but I didn't. My marriage fell apart in 1974. I went to live at the "Low Life Motel" for a couple of years after Jean and I broke up. The divorce was about all I could handle if I was handling it. For some reason, my life fell apart all at once, but medicine never gave up on me.

The divorced men I knew said I had it wrong. Still, I needed to talk to someone who'd been through a divorce, and I didn't want to talk to a woman yet. I saw only trouble there in case I gave myself away and got in too deep. So, I played it safe and hung out with the guys. "So, your marriage failed; welcome to the club. That's what marriages do. Lighten up. Look at it like this."

I'd be fine after psychotherapy. Once you find your destiny and embrace a plan for "emotional growth," you're halfway home, and getting there is half the fun. Think of the sex. Women in LA love sensitive guys who know something about emotional growth, guys who read books and go to lectures, guys with decent catch phrases. Hell, listen to us. Yeah, listen to them. They might have well have said, "Don't worry about death. It's over once you're through it."

"You can wimp and whine all you want. But if you're getting laid enough, you don't care what happened to your marriage, a dumb idea in the first place. LA is the place to be. We're the envy of married guys the world over, don't you see?"

Yeah, maybe so. Still, it seemed a lot like a contagion might get worse before it got better. I knew some diseases like that, and plenty of them were going around. Maybe that was my nature. Whatever the crowd said was right, I didn't believe. Whatever the trend was, I didn't trust it. That's how I was in my medical practice by then. I didn't buy the latest gadgets, procedures, or conclusions any more. The medical professor I revered and accompanied to the Winnebago Indian Reservation once said to me after we'd studied an inconclusive paper on cholesterol and coronary heart disease, though the authors tried to make it sound conclusive. "You're a lot like me. So, be neither the first nor the last on the bandwagon."

Maybe that's why I was struggling. Practicing medicine didn't make you better at practicing life. As a physician, you knew your patient's pain alright, but do you know yours? In those days, I felt responsible for what had gone wrong in the marriage. The guilt that came from failure, the guilt that came from knowing you could have done more if you were paying attention, if you weren't so busy becoming somebody.

The "Low Life" was south of Santa Monica Boulevard, not the best part of West LA; no prestigious zip code here, though the city had a handful. They told people where you lived, what you did, and who you thought you were. The sign out front said "The Hanford Arms," as if you were sitting down to a spot of tea in Yorkshire or Cornwall.

The Hanford Arms must have been a two-story motel at one time though no one else seemed to know or care. The diagonal parking spaces next to the building had alternating numbers on them indicating one "apartment" on the ground level and another above. I reasoned that the studio apartment next to the curb had been the office in the motel's heyday. I lived in 11A on the ground floor. Mr. Chen and his family lived just above me in 21A.

Still, we had outdoor plants next to the studio or the office, depending on your take. I had no idea who'd put them in or who took care of them, but they were there, our little rays of sunshine. Some lived in a wooden trough under the office window sill, mums and geraniums. Below, a metal trough suspended by wires held jade plants and cactuses, more robust than the mums and geraniums. To be useful on the premises, I bought a watering can in case any of them needed me.

I didn't know my neighbors either, but we smiled a lot in passing. Lacking fluency in Spanish or Chinese, I had little to say. My strength in high school had been Latin, and in college, German. I did come to know Mr. Chen, though our chats were short once he knew I was a doctor. I was a mark after that.

We'd run into each other heading to work in the morning. He was a wiry fellow, probably five-foot-three-inches tall and maybe a hundred and twenty pounds soaking wet. As best I could tell, he was a bit of a con artist with a deal a day for me. He spoke what was then called "pidgin English," now "Chinglish." When he got to his point after a few limp phrases, his left eyelid sagged, as if done in by the effort. It gave away his agenda too, not what you'd call a normal wink. We shared nothing intimate in those moments. "So, you doctor, huh? Two things if OK for you right now. You already, huh, now for me?" Wink.

In a way, he was my mother, a preening cat, a crafty survivor in a world he thought he knew but didn't. And nothing was about to stop them.

Looking back on it, he put two deals on the table. Did I want his 1956 Oldsmobile 98 or was I interested in his daughter, a twenty-year old physical therapy student in Santa Monica? I'd seen the "Olds,' an ocean liner, five miles a gallon on its best days, and we had a gasoline crisis in LA. And I'd seen Mimi, exquisite, like Nancy Kwan in the film version of "Flower Drum Song" by Rodgers and Hammerstein. That part of the bargain I'd see if the ocean liner weren't in on the deal, but I doubted he'd deliver. Most likely, Mimi had other ideas.

———

The apartment I was looking at two years later on Wellesley Avenue was in a neighborhood from 1910 or so. The building was too old and quaint to have been a motel, and it was a half block north of Wilshire Boulevard on a street lined with azalea shrubs and palm trees. Bougainvillea vines showed off the Spanish-styled houses. Some had yellow flowers, others white, and still others, magenta. I was smitten. The landlord mentioned "the prestigious 90049 zip code" the day I saw the place. I was eager to come up in the world. Maybe he had me pegged.

The second bedroom would be a Godsend when the kids were with me. The kitchen was spacious with a walk-in pantry jutting off. A back door opened onto a little terrace leading to a staircase below. The terrace was big enough for a table to have a meal on or maybe a barbecue would fit there. A sense of normalcy was setting in. The furniture must have come from odd lots at garage sales. Greenish-brown serpiginous stains were scattered on the carpet. Never mind, the furniture could be arranged. I liked the place.

The best part was a neighbor who threw herself into the fray. A vivacious elderly German widow vowed to look after me as "the son she'd never had." She lived across the courtyard in the next building. Slender, elegant in her look, breezy and eloquent in her English, she'd met an American army captain of German descent. He brought her to the States in 1949. Two years later, her husband died in his late thirties of a malignant brain tumor. For over a month, he'd smelled natural gas wherever he went and was dead six weeks later. Frau Feldman didn't marry again.

Her story brought to mind my beloved George Gershwin, who'd died of a malignant brain tumor, a glioblastoma multiforme, the worst cancer you can imagine. By the time you know you have it, you might as well be dead. Gershwin went numb at the piano moments into the second movement of his "Concerto in F." The San Francisco Symphony Orchestra was thrown off kilter. He picked it up, and they finished the piece with a flourish, but he must have been in agony, wondering what was wrong. Later offstage, when his brother asked him, George said, "I don't know, Ira. I smelled burnt rubber, sulfur, or something. I couldn't find the keys for a few seconds."

An olfactory hallucination, a false smell due to a tumor in the temporal lobe on one side of his brain, did him in. False smells killed just about anyone who had them for long. He was gone in two weeks at thirty-eight. The music world and the rest of us never knew or heard his mature genius. Life is precious and fleeting, whether you're famous or not. Frau Feldman's husband had met a similar fate.

"Doctors are so dedicated and work so hard; and the children, your children are so precious! I love them. Come live with us. We're good people," she said.

How could I resist her? She was fresh air. She had convictions though I didn't share them all. "Some doctors are and some aren't; some do and some don't," I thought. Dedicated to what and working hard for what reason were my questions. There were doctors, and there were doctors. That's how my mind worked then, an odd time of no absolute truths. Everything was open to question. But my children were precious; she had that right. And I knew some German from college; that's all I had, some phrases like Mr. Chen's pidgin English. My Latin was stronger than my German, but I never winked at her as if my left eyelid had given out.

"*Guten Tag* or *Danke schoen,* Frau Feldman," I'd say. We became fast friends after I moved in. Before then, I worried I'd miss Mr. Chen, or maybe more, Mimi gliding by my window on her platform shoes on the way up to 21A. I decided to rent on Wellesley anyway. I knew how to find the "Low Life," and I knew when the two of them would be around.

———

When I made my first run to a coin-operated laundry on Wilshire Boulevard at the corner of Barrington Avenue, the 90049 zip code let me down. A young man lay in his vomit in front of the dryers. I wondered how long he'd been there and whether anyone had tried to help. As I came closer, he woke up, rolled over and, in a foggy state, asked to borrow three dollars for the bus fare to the Veterans Administration Hospital in Sepulveda, an hour away by telephone in the San Fernando Valley. His name was Paul. When I told him that the Wadsworth VA Hospital was only a few blocks up the road, he knew and didn't want to go there.

Wadsworth was a jewel then, the flagship in the VA Healthcare System on manicured grounds with its own zip code, 90073. The hospital building was new. An airy atrium, the elegant lobby, and foliage dangling from the balconies made you think you'd wandered into a Hyatt Regency Hotel by mistake until you saw sixty feet of "Old Glory" draped from ceiling to floor at the back of the foyer.

The flagship hadn't done him much good. He didn't want anything to do with it, and he cursed me, railing about a lawsuit. His hands trembled finely, and his limbs shook coarsely. He wore a band on his wrist from Wadsworth after signing out "against medical advice." I assumed his problem was alcohol or drug use, a Vietnam veteran, I guessed from his age. I'd cared for many at the VA Hospital in Seattle. When I looked into his eyes, full of emptiness and drowning in need, I worried about my eight- year-old son, Michael.

Here Paul was, every parent's nightmare, and here was that damned fear of losing your son to a toxic world you couldn't control. He didn't want to go back to Wadsworth, but he'd be better off there than in a hospital where no one knew him. I gave him a dollar and pushed him onto the bus after talking to the driver. "Can you make sure he goes into the VA after he gets off the bus? They'll recognize him and know what to do.'

"I don't have time, behind on my route."

"OK. Give me a second to start the laundry. I'll walk back, just in time to put my clothes in the dryer."

"It's OK, Doc, if you feel that strong about it. I'll get him in with help from the passengers. The bus goes right by the emergency entrance."

Zip codes gave us no wisdom in a toxic society, no guidance for little ones. The rot that gave parents nightmares could be in the neighborhood before you woke up in the morning. Maybe they're working on a vaccine. That's how I saw it then, but I didn't know shit about social sciences.

———

The first few weeks in the new apartment were up and down in a rhythm I came to expect but didn't relish. Frau Feldman was a rock in my life. My children loved her, and I needed her grace.

Jean and I had separated in no hurry for a divorce. I supported the family while she finished college, but the finances were in trouble. I had minor pay increases at the University Hospital though I was doing the poorest work of my young career. No patients suffered. My clinical skill was a given now after years of rigorous training; taking care of patients is what kept me sane.

Research in the laboratory was another story, needing a creativity I couldn't muster. When I grappled with the herpes virus I worked on (cytomegalovirus), my focus was gone in a bang, like air blasting out of a pricked balloon. It was a deceitful little critter though it was huge as viruses went. Big in other ways too, in structure, complicated in its genetics, and confusing in its replication. I blamed my pager for going off with calls from doctors and patients when I couldn't follow its footprints. After the interruptions, I'd go back to the well, but it was still dry. At times, I thought the damned virus had betrayed me after giving me a reputation of sorts early in my career.

I knew all about clinical research, microbiology, and the epidemiology of infectious diseases, but I didn't know much about basic disease mechanisms or how to get at them. The scientific grounding I needed to reach that goal wasn't mine yet; that's why I was at the University Hospital on a short leash in Dr. Steven Jackson's laboratory.

I believed in the path I'd chosen, though few of my peers had taken it. To me, it was the highest calling in medicine. I knew I was a fine doctor. But I wanted more, to leave a legacy to the field that had called me, the field I'd called my own. I wanted to be at the forefront, to find the truth, and to mentor young physicians with that passion. Together, we'd take knowledge from the laboratory bench to the patient's bedside; we'd have insight into how these damned diseases really worked and what the virus did to cause all this misery. We'd be tough on ourselves and on our experimental data. And, we'd agree to make less money as part of the deal. But maybe, it was a naïve dream or an overly generous estimate of my ability.

I thought about private practice for the first time. Then, I could focus on patient care with no research to fret over and only a little teaching to do. The siren's call was heard. Yeah, I admit it now; I was tempted to ditch my lofty goal "to give new knowledge to the field that called me." The temptation pained me most when I gave a research lecture to a group of private physicians. The medical licensing board mandated that community physicians had to attend a certain number of scientific lectures a year. I hated giving them. Their eyes glazed over, and their heads bobbed up and down trying to stay awake. "Yeah, yeah," they were thinking if they were thinking. "Is this virus important to *my* practice? If so, tell me what to do. Otherwise, I don't want to hear about it." Hell, I hadn't suggested the topic for this lecture. Someone else, one of them, had.

They had a point. I didn't know what to do about it either. At times, I knew my future might be brighter if I were one of them, a "schmoozer," looking for smiles, handshakes, and patient referrals. Then, I could sit back and doze off whenever a blowhard with his shitty salary from the University came over to give greedy heathens his take on how to practice medicine. Let him go on about a virus you couldn't treat. I'd have the hours of "Continuing Medical Education" I need to renew my medical license. Come back and see us when we can do something about the damned virus. Neither side had any idea what the other had to put up with. For now, I stayed the course.

———

The dreams came on in spring, 1977. I hadn't remembered a dream in years. Why they came on all of a sudden, I don't know, maybe a kind of twisted wake-up call. They frightened me with their vivid edginess and a sense of urgency. I'd wake up in the night, doused in sweat, my heart pounding. What happened in the dream and my reaction to it was "out of synch." They weren't nightmares, just pernicious barbed wires ripping away at my mind and soul. I'd never dreamt about endless falls or an inability to run from danger that friends had described. Yet I knew the dreams were on a quest, convoluted maybe, but they wanted something.

In the first one, Jean and I, our children, and a man Jean was dating then rode in my car to our house in Pacific Palisades, a coastal suburb west of Los Angeles. We were all in the back seat except for the driver. The car shut down at the curb three houses too soon. Getting out, I saw that Angela, my nine-year-old daughter was driving. That's why we'd stopped too soon.

Once in the house on a mission, I sorted through drawers and cabinets looking for meaning. My secretary at the hospital walked in holding a faded newspaper she thought was important. Stock market summaries filled one page; they meant nothing to me. On the second page, a beaming new mother in her hospital bed held the "first baby of the New Year," the headline said. Now, I was animated, nearly hysterical, asking my secretary if she thought the baby were me. No, she didn't think so. "Look at the date on it," she said. The date was April 4, 1913.

Jean's boyfriend wanted me in the kitchen. Why I'd first met him, I didn't see why she was attracted. In the dream, though, he was handsome and decisive; he was seduction and potency. He crouched under the sink with muscles rippling and pointed at pipes. He said with gritty emphasis how surprised he was that the plumbing was so shoddy, especially since the man who owned this house was said to be a master craftsman. The shortcuts were obvious to anyone who knew where to look.

Who the hell is he, and what is he doing in our kitchen after I'd put in two years at the "Low Life?" He's inspecting the plumbing, without being asked, in the house I pay the mortgage on? Maybe you should worry about your own plumbing, Mr. Potency. There isn't a damned thing wrong with mine, I'll tell you that.

But I knew too that it wasn't strictly a sexual metaphor. The message pointed to a core I needed to find again, the sooner, the better.

I expected to hear more now from my subconscious after years of nothing. In the morning, the lyrics of a popular song by Cat Stevens rumbled through my head just as the verse shifted to the refrain:

"Did it take long to find me? I asked the fateful light.

Did it take long to find me, and are you gonna stay the night?"

Then back to the verse:

"Oh, I'm bein' followed by a moon shadow, moon shadow, moon shadow, oh, oh."

Though I didn't know it that morning, April 4, 1913 was my dead father's date of birth. He'd say so the day I met him six months later at lunch in a pub near his home in Leicester, England. I've never figured out how the hell I knew this. My mother might have told me, but I doubt it. After we came to America in 1947, she wanted to obliterate every vestige of our past in England.

———

The second dream came a few nights later. I was on a hike. A lush and oddly pale grass covered the hills and valleys. This must be Scotland, I remember thinking. The sheep on the slope didn't mind me hiking by. A thick mist hung over the hill's crests as ancient stone walls three feet high cut the fields below into a ragged quilt. I heard music now and then. A plaintive violin melody had me proud and sad with its notes soaring and plunging. Higher up, smoke wafted from the chimney of a stone cottage. The music, so familiar and so foreign, was coming from it. When I was nearly there, I broke into a run, laughing, giddy like a child. Suddenly, a pack of snarling dogs with flashing teeth surrounded me. I stopped quiet after the commotion and saw the door to the cottage open. An old man in a kilt held the doorway. He had thick gray hair and an unkempt beard. With an ax in his right hand and a shovel in his left, he had work to do. At least, that's what I hoped they were for. He said, riveting his gaze on me, his hazel eyes my own. "So then, y'ave come, 'ave ye? You're here at last?"

He was angry. As I moved closer to explain the trespassing, the dogs pulled back, giving in to him. I knew he was my father, my dead father. He was here alright, but I wasn't welcome. Yes, he'd have years on him now, wouldn't he, if he'd survived that beach in Normandy?

The dreams wanted me to take up a past I'd denied, it seemed. But would they stand by me? I trusted them to an extent and, each morning, I wrote them down in as much detail as I could remember. Was I wrong to trust them? Maybe so, but if I couldn't trust what came from within, who or what the hell else was there? A journey was on whether or not I liked it. I wasn't sure I was ready for the ride.

————

That night, after a glass of wine, I set off on a promenade through the neighborhood I'd neglected. Frau Feldman waved me a send off. After a month in charge of a medical ward, I savored my freedom, sleeping in a bit tomorrow, and turning off the pager. The evening was stunning as it cooled. The unpretentious houses and well-kept gardens charmed me. I hadn't thought this possible in Los Angeles, maybe the benefits of "the prestigious 90049 zip code." Old people lived here. Bless them and their noble lives, having raised families for decades. They dwelt everyday on a goldmine unknown to them while realtors lay quietly alert for the inevitable, like vultures scheming on a clothes-line in the backyard.

Gregarious, I stopped to chat with neighbors trimming roses and shrubs or tending bougainvillea. As I strolled on, the neighborhood was more vivid than I'd expected. The sky at sunset was lustrous with streaky, linear gray clouds veiling a lower portion of the sun. At a corner, I saw an old man rocking in a chair on his porch.

He'd closed his eyes, his face wrinkled and serenely weathered. The chair took him back and forth in its rhythm. Though I was within feet of him, he didn't wake up. As I stood there, his uniqueness made my heart beat faster. The man was perfect and beautiful. No man exactly like him existed. The impish expression on his face said so and told you to go to hell if you didn't believe it.

The perfect man rocked away. What a silly world I'd lived in. Every person, tree, or flower is perfect, not too short, too broad, existing as it can. Damn it, and damn the time wasted wishing for something or someone a little better. All things are perfect in that they are as they should be, as God intended them. I was the one who'd not seen the beauty.

My reverie gave me a glance at a world I didn't know. Just as I thought I might soar, the pain was intense, the blunt trauma of loss. My revelation slipped away, and I couldn't sustain it. Slumping on the porch, holding my forehead in my hand, tears fell. The old man was still sleeping, unaware of his perfection.

I don't know how long I sat there, minutes to half-an-hour. My pal was lapping away, serene as ever. No one came to arrest me for violating the premises. "Reality" was back, and I needed to make a call to ask a question with a "yes or no" answer. How hard should that be? Still, I dreaded asking it.

———

I sat on the couch, heels propped up in slippers on a glass-topped blue coffee table, probably one of many colors in its history. I was pensive; no, that wasn't the way to put it. Worse than that, I was brooding. Something was wrong with how I'd lived my life. I wasn't connected to simple joys, the pleasures of being and seeing. I was dutifully fortified, at times impregnable. My mind was boggy with evaluations and estimations, interpretations and calculations. Now, I knew why. To be naïve, innocent, vulnerable, to breath in the world without a filter, brought devastation after the joy.

Thoughts drifted to my mother. What the hell had happened to the Nora who'd laughed and tickled me as we listened to "Amos and Andy" Sunday nights on the radio? She knew how much I loved her then because I'd told her. That was before whatever happened to her happened, before she went missing, unaccountable to me or anyone else for the rest of her life. One day, she disappeared as the mother I loved and returned as a stranger I didn't know and didn't want to know.

What was the evidence my father was dead? Everything had come from Nora. No one else had ever mentioned his death; not my grandparents, not my mother's brother Peter, and not even my stepfather. Why was that? Were they protecting me from something, grief? Not likely. If my father were dead, they'd have referred to his death or celebrated his life now and again, wouldn't they? I didn't even know if he was in the Infantry, the Royal Air Force, or the Royal Navy. How stupid of me as a student of World War II precisely because my father had been killed in the conflict. And where were the details of his life? There weren't any.

I tried to cling to a story woven into my childhood. But the return of my longing for him wouldn't let me get away with it. I was aware I was letting a cruel hoax go, but I struggled to release it. I was like mercury oozing out of a broken thermometer, the quicksilver I'd played with as a kid. One minute it was consistent and trustworthy; the next fragmented and elusive. But it was never what you wanted it to be.

Then, there were the dreams, the baby in the newspaper born on April 4, 1913, an old man brandishing a shovel and an axe in the Scottish Highlands to haunting violin music. I thought I'd seen him again rocking on a porch up the street tonight.

If someone had spoken of my father, who would've spoken? Obviously, not my mother. And I'd been out of touch with Aunt Amelia and Uncle Peter in England for decades. Oddly, my stepfather had never mentioned my father. Did Bert Jordan believe that my father had been killed, deluded by Nora? It wouldn't surprise me. Or was there collusion between them, maybe at Nora's insistence, to nurture a lie? No matter what, Bert was the curator and the sole potential donor of the truth. Where the hell had I been all these years?

"Do you have a listing for a Bert L. Jordan in Orange County, operator? The first name is spelled B-E-R-T, not B-U-R-T." I was really Bertram, Bertram Lee, I remembered that all of a sudden as if it were yesterday; funny how memory was so acute tonight after decades of fog. I hadn't seen or spoken to Bert in twenty years. Had he remarried as my mother had heard? Was he still in Orange County? How would he react to my call? "714-961-4430," thank you, operator."

I put ice cubes in a glass and poured a short scotch. I hadn't had whiskey in years and was surprised that I had any. I wanted to call, but I was fearful. I remembered ugly hateful scenes between this man and my mother when I was a boy. The separation and divorce had been volatile. As I nursed the drink, I dug up some bravado. I didn't care how Bert reacted. I just wanted to ask a question. How tough should that be?

"Hello, Bert."

"Yeah,"

"How are you? It's Colin." He responded with a muffled sigh.

"I'm sorry to bother you. I want to ask you something."

"That's fine, Colin, just so you know I don't need anything to do with your mother again. Don't tell her you found me."

"Yes, I know. How've you been?"

"I'm fine and married happy now. I have two sons, eleven and eight, and I'm still working in the oil fields. I'm a foreman."

"Good for you. I see you're still in Orange County. I'd like to see you."

"I have no objection. Just don't tell her where I am. Everything's going good now."

"No. Don't worry. I'm a doctor, Bert, on the faculty at the University Hospital in LA."

I was calling him "Bert" rather than "Dad" for the first time in my life.

"So, you really did make it, huh?"

It hadn't occurred to me I'd "made it," but I'd gotten somewhere. Where I was going from here was what worried me. "I guess so. After medical school, I did an internship and residency at the University of Washington in Seattle with a couple of years in the service mixed in."

"Well, congratulations. I always wondered what happened to you."

"Bert, there's something I need to ask. I hope you don't mind. It's about my father. My mother has always claimed he was killed in the war, right? Well, I'm asking you now point blank. Is it true?"

After a pause of about fifteen seconds, I heard nothing on the other end. What was he thinking? What had he known all these years? "Bert?"

"Shit, Colin, I can't believe it. She's still saying that? You mean she hasn't told you?"

"Told me what?"

"He's not dead as far as I know. I never met the man, but I know he came home to England after the war. He had some reputation as a soldier and, I think, he must have been decorated. He was living in the same area, somewhere near Dukinfield."

I bolted up. The chair toppled over and crashed into a plant stand. The pot shattered on the floor. I couldn't speak, I couldn't breathe. I don't know what I said to Bert after that, but I hoped I was civil and thankful in my "good bye." Lightheaded, I nearly fainted. At first wanting to keep the peace between my mother and me, my thought was "She's a cunning little thing, isn't she?" But then, I roared "Damn the bitch. I knew it! She had no right. For Christ's sake, I have a father, and he's alive!"

———

At midnight, I put in another call, still sipping the scotch, brooding less. I needed a phone number in England. Let's hope he's still there, still alive, alive the way he was when I was a lad.

"Yes, that's right operator, Peter Glynn in Dukinfield, United Kingdom. It's a small town in Cheshire."

"One moment, sir. United States calling, operator, the overseas information code for Mr. Peter Glynn – G-L-Y-N-N, Dukinfield, Cheshire, United Kingdom."

When she came on, the British operator's voice calmed me with its familiar lilt. My mind was on a cobblestone street, a cotton mill, and a canal where my cousins John and Nat and I launched toy sailboats to one another. We'd play "hide and seek" and "kick the can" in churchyards turned to rubble by the bombing, spend an afternoon in the hills "train spotting," and then go to afternoon tea with Aunt Amelia and Uncle Peter. "Hello, have I reached Mr. Peter Glynn?"

"Yes, 'tis he. Good morning to you. But who are you? You're not calling from this country."

"Uncle Peter, this is Colin in America. How are you? ……Peter it's……

"Colin, my God!"

"Sorry to hit you out of the blue, but I don't have your address. How's Aunt Amelia?"

"She's champion. It's incredible to hear you speak as an adult! You've lost your British accent for some bloody reason. Excuse me…… I'm a bit overwhelmed. Is Nora well?"

Oh, he was alive alright. His wit and his heart were still mine. I said in a quaking voice, "My mother's fine, and John and Nat?"

"John moved to South Africa a year ago. He works for a chemist's firm, International Pharmaceuticals Limited. I believe they're quite well-known in your country. Nat's a brewer at Tollys, the largest beer company in England. Bloody hell, Colin! It's nearly eight in the morning. I'm just leaving for work to do some welding. What time is it there?"

"It's midnight. I need your help in tracking down my father. I want to come over as soon as I can."

"Amelia, Amelia! Our cheeky nephew in America is calling after all these years. What nerve the little bugger has! He's coming over to look for Mitchell Colville. Suddenly, it's top priority!"

"Colin, I haven't seen him in nearly thirty years; yes, just after the war, 1948 in Oldham. I ran into his brother Jack a couple of years ago. He owns a manufacturing concern there. Jack will know where to reach him. What's your address? By way, I'll enclose a note for Nora. She owes me a few bloody good letters!"

"Thanks, Uncle Peter. I appreciate your help. It'll be wonderful to see you both."

"You know Colin what our last memory is of you? The day you left for America when you spilled apples onto the tracks beneath the train! Do you remember that awful morning?"

"Yes, I do. I love you, and I can't wait to see you." I had to get off the phone.

After we'd hung up, emotion broke out, and I sobbed for half-an-hour. I couldn't tell whether the tears came from guilt or the joy of reconciliation. Once again, I was that lad of six on his way to board a ship called the Queen Elizabeth in Southampton. My mum had said "it's a city that floats across the sea, the Atlantic Ocean to New York." To get to Southampton, we had to take a train from Manchester. I was carrying a bag of apples, though I didn't know why. After all, they must have apples in New York and America, mustn't they? Maybe they gave me something to do, an assignment of sorts. A few spilled out of my sack onto the tracks at the train station. Irritated at my clumsiness and lack of responsibility, I jumped down to retrieve them. Several had bounced between the iron wheels of the train's steam engine. The train had twelve massive wheels much taller than I was, I remember that, and the departure whistle was screeching with deafening intensity. At six, I wasn't frightened. After all, I'd been through the bombing. As I tried to get farther under the engine, an adult took my arms and lifted me back onto the platform.

One last apple spilled out of my sack. I don't know who rescued me, but it must have been Uncle Peter, my mother, or Bert Jordan.

I'd shared nothing of this in America. In recent years, I'd had few close friends, just colleagues who'd never heard about it. I was shocked tonight. Thirty years had gone with little thought of my family in England, and few thoughts at all of a father who, of course, had been killed in war. My mother didn't encourage questions, but what about my neglect?

As a child, I'd adored my aunt and uncle, and I'd never had chums like John and Nat in America. We were brothers, and their parents were mine. A naïve lad, worried about all the wrong things, had spilled apples under a screeching steam engine on his way to board a city that sailed the sea.

———

The next morning, a Saturday, I set off for Santa Monica, a beach town west of the University Medical Center. A community of ex-patriot Brits lived here. Some of them were my patients, and some of them believed that my father had been killed on a beach in Normandy. I was headed to the public library.

I had energy to burn after the phone calls last night. More than that, I was manic. I wanted to put the energy to use before I found out how tired I was from the month on service. I needed to cut loose a ruthless spy for investigative work I could sink my teeth into.

"Do you have a section of phone books from the United Kingdom?"

"Yes we do. It's very popular, just up the stairs to the left, sir."

I wanted my father's phone number though I had no reason to think I'd find it. And I didn't. I tried the county Cheshire, but pages had been torn out. I knew my father's family was from Scotland, but nothing either in Glasgow or Edinburgh. In Oldham, where uncle Peter had said my father's brother Jack lived, I did find a listing for a "Jack Colville." But when I called the listing the next morning, the man was not related my father.

When I got out of the car at my apartment after the library, Frau Feldman was holding court between the buildings. Radiant in a flowery sun dress, she was gliding in elegance on the flagstone, combing the premises.

"I heard a crash and shouting in your place last night. The windows were open. I was watering plants outside. I was worried, but you looked OK when I got a glimpse of you – just a bit agitated. Maybe you'd like to come over tonight for a glass of riesling or gewürztraminer cold on my patio?"

I took her up on it in favor of gewürztraminer. Once I was on the patio, a rusty plug forced its way through the faucet, and it all poured out about my mother, my stepfather, my aunt and uncle in England, my cousins, my life there, my life here, the bombing, my marriage, and what I didn't know about my father.

"Destiny's calling. Be patient, be strong. I can't imagine anything like that. You have to seize the moment. I wish I had."

I didn't want destiny. I wanted to change the subject after the raw show I'd put on.

"Oh, I know you can imagine it. Tell me about you and your husband."

She was startled at my probing, but settled down as if knowing my intent.

"It's about Jews. Does that interest you?"

"Sure it does if it's about you."

She sighed and folded her hands in her lap as if she wasn't sure she should tell me. Then her face flushed.

"I'm guilty of a crime, a crime called cowardice."

"I don't believe you. What do you mean?"

"When I was a girl in Germany, my name was Feldman as it is now, a Jewish name because we were Jews. My father was worried when the Nazis were coming to power. He changed the name to "Fiedler," which isn't Jewish. In German, it means "fiddler." He was making a clever play on "Fiddler on the Roof." I had no brothers the Nazis could check for circumcision, but it drove me crazy when the SS troops rounded up our people for the camps. No justice, no recourse. I sobbed when they left. They knew our name had been changed, and they could have turned us in, but they didn't. I couldn't look them in the eye when they were taken off. I've been racked with guilt ever since."

"You aren't guilty of anything! Your father was protecting his family and did a damned good job. Hell, he should've lied to the bastards."

I don't know if she heard me. Tears were all over her face. Then, she gave out her hands, and I took them. Her eyes were still closed.

"I'm glad you came over tonight. I've never told anyone except my husband."

"Hilda, tell me about him."

She sighed a moment and then responded as it were about time someone had asked.

"His name is Ernest Zimmerman. I talk to him every night. He's a reformed Jew from Los Angeles. His family is German. He's fluent in English, German, and Hebrew, witty and smart. He can imitate anyone – Oliver Hardy, Jack Benny, Ed Burns, or Groucho Marx. He's handsome. He's…..he was…..a damned good Jew and a fine man. He didn't mind when I refused to change my name to Zimmerman. I wanted Feldman, but now I wonder."

She started to sob, and I took her in my arms. I don't know how long she cried. I was off kilter. I guess we both were, but the gewürztraminer wasn't the reason. She found her footing. With fire in her eyes, she blurted out. "Why is life like this, so damned hard? I miss Ernest. It wasn't fair what happened to him. My last thought is the fucking gas smells he complained about. My only consolation is that gas didn't get him in Auschwitz, and, more recently, your story about George Gershwin."

After I said goodnight and crossed the courtyard, Hilda Feldman and Ernest Zimmerman were on my mind. Another Jew, Paul Simon had put it best in "Bookends."

"Preserve your memories. They're all that's left you."

———

In those days, I was intent on atoning for my neglect wherever I found it. When I left for medical school, I kept in touch with Dr. Ellen Hawkins, sending a Christmas card and a personal note each year. But once I started internship and residency, I let them drop, probably because I was overwhelmed with training and family life. A few days after speaking to Uncle Peter, I called her office. "Hi, it's Dr. Colin Jordan at the University Hospital in LA. Do you know if Dr. Hawkins has time to come to the phone or maybe to call me back?"

"Are you the Colin Jordan who used to come to the clinic and go on rounds?"

"Yes."

"Just a moment. I'll get her partner, Dr. Dixon. You remember her, don't you?"

"Yes, of course, I remember Angie."

Something was wrong, and my heart sank. I braced myself. Oh please God, don't let Ellen be dead.

"Hi Colin! We've followed your progress, and we were delighted when the University Hospital said in the bulletin that you'd joined the faculty. I loved your paper on salmonella and that damned meat slicer. Your work on CMV has been impressive, but tough for us to understand. Anyway, we're proud in Orange County. Congratulations."

"Thanks, Angie. I had no idea you knew about it. But I'm scared to ask, is Ellen alright?"

"She's fine, but refuses the call because you're an ingrate. She's fuming at her desk."

I pulled myself together. "Ellen's right. That's why I called. I'm an ingrate in the old country too. Here's my home phone and pager at the University Hospital. I'd love to hear from you."

Ellen called me at home that night. "Sorry to bust your balls, but I've been pissed at you for years."

"Sorry I neglected you, no excuses. Can we go back to square one, Ellen?"

"We're proud of what you've done and our little part in it. I was delighted you went into infectious diseases. That's what I'd have done if I'd gone into internal medicine or pediatrics. Would you mind if one of us came up for infectious disease rounds from time to time, kind of like a role reversal?"

"Christ, are you kidding, a role reversal? You taught me more in three months than I could teach either of you in ten years. I'll send you the attending physician schedule so you know when I'm on call. And I'll tell the rest of the faculty to expect you if you want to come up any other time. Thanks for the call, Ellen. I'll look forward to seeing you. I'm sorry."

CHAPTER 8

SENORA CISNEROS AND A FILM STUDIO

"Senora Cisneros has disseminated tuberculosis," I announced as the attending physician on the internal medicine ward, trying to fire up the medical students. Two of them, on call the night before, were dozing off while another presented the patient's history and physical. The team wasn't expecting bombast. Still, as a third-year student, you don't sleep through attending rounds on internal medicine, the clerkship most likely to define what you'll do.

I held court now, certain of the diagnosis. I relished being in charge, as long as it lasted, the familiar haven of clinical medicine, my sanctuary. At least here, I was sane, and a dream wouldn't come barging in.

"Tuberculosis pulls it all together. She's had fever and low blood counts for three months, and now her liver functions are abnormal. The lymph nodes in her abdomen are swollen on the scans. We can't miss the diagnosis because it's treatable. She could have leukemia or a lymphoma too early to diagnose, but I don't think so. Even if I'm wrong, surgery will tell us. Let's ask the surgeons to see her for an abdominal exploration. We have to find out what's in those lymph nodes. I know you're tired of hearing me say it, but nothing takes the place of a diagnosis."

"What about her low platelet count? I don't see tuberculosis causing that. Plus, she'd risk uncontrollable bleeding during surgery."

Dr. David Miller was an inquisitive senior resident in internal medicine. He'd been at the top of his class at Michigan, but he wasn't with me on this one. He was sullen, argumentative this morning. Maybe the night on call had been a rough go.

"David, the kind of tuberculosis I'm worried about often causes low platelet counts. That's a reason to suspect it here. As for bleeding, we'll give her platelets during surgery. The surgeons may be reluctant to operate, but we have to convince them we need a diagnosis. We can't commit her to a year of treatment for tuberculosis without it. The drugs are too toxic to justify the risk. Surgery is the only way to find out what she has. The only other choice we've got is to fiddle around, testing forever, until we break the bank."

"I know you're pushing Sutton's Law, but I've never seen tuberculosis show up like this. I'm not sure we should be *so* aggressive. She's awfully fragile."

Bless him. He was right.

"David, yes, she's fragile, and she'll be more fragile as every day goes by. We have to do it now while we can."

I pulled back in my chair to rethink it, taking in his objection.

"Old fashioned tuberculosis" shows up like this time and again, not the form we see nowadays in the lungs. Every kind of abnormal blood count happens when it involves the bone marrow and the lymph nodes. The bone marrow exam didn't help us, and we have nowhere else to go. It's at the top of the list as a cause of unexplained fever. Plus she's from Mexico. Come on! Let's all go in and see her."

"Senora Cisneros, we've looked into your tests, and we think you have an unusual form of tuberculosis, one that's tough to diagnose. It's in the lymph glands in your abdomen, your belly. I'm afraid you'll need surgery to be sure. If it is tuberculosis, we can treat it with drugs after the operation."

"Tuberculosis! Am I contagious? Have my children or husband gotten it from me?"

She was elegant, lovely, a matriarch in speech and gesture. Her hair was up in the way Eva Peron and Esperanza in Albuquerque wore theirs, and she had make-up on, not common on this ward. The team must have told her the attending physician would be in to see her this morning. Her husband and children knew she'd stand up to any news that came along to protect them all. Her English was strong and clear. Everything about her was. She enthralled me.

David stood discreetly behind me, holding back a smirk. "Let Jordan take the brunt of this," I guessed he was thinking. "After all, he's the attending physician, the doctor responsible for whatever goes wrong."

It wasn't so much that I was a mind-reader. I just knew how I felt as a resident when the attending physician went off the deep end like this, gambling on a diagnosis "to pull it all together" in a Petersdorf-like maneuver. OK, I admit it; the 'Dorf may have colored my judgment with his theatrics.

David wouldn't be party to false hope. He wouldn't take a journey to find the balm of Gilead to heal her as I read him. The medical students were shocked and confused, tuberculosis indeed. They didn't believe this poor woman, who clearly had leukemia, was about to be tormented by risky and unnecessary surgery.

"It's not a kind of tuberculosis that's contagious because it's not in your lungs, at least not yet," I went on, looking into her eyes, needing her support for her own good. "Tuberculosis wouldn't be a bad disease for you. We have treatment, but it needs a long course, probably a year in your case. That's why we need surgery to be sure we have it right." I didn't say anything about the side effects of the drugs. I'd bring them up when the time came.

Mrs. Cisneros wanted closure. Now, her tearful eyes betrayed her bravado. "You mean I *don't* have leukemia? I've been worried about it. I even discussed it with my family to get them ready in case I don't come home."

The hope in the question, and the way she'd posed it stunned me. Leukemia, my God. "I don't think so. Leukemia can start out like this, but I think tuberculosis is much more likely. Why are you worried about leukemia?"

"Oh, one of your doctors mentioned it to me."

My neck must have gone crimson as I bent over, holding her hand. I knew my face had. Who'd said "leukemia," for Christ's sake? And what kind of leukemia did the idiot think she had? Sure, leukemia was in the running, but you don't say that to a patient until the evidence is under a microscope. I suspected David. "Mrs. Cisneros, you don't have leukemia. We'd never advise an operation you didn't need."

Her eyes flashed a glimmer of hope to me. Demurring, she said. "Whatever you think is best, doctor. I trust you."

Maybe her blind faith would turn sour if I were wrong. Still, she had to trust me even if the team didn't. I wanted to take her in my arms. I held her hand instead, trying to show her that we were on the same side. "We're conservative about surgery. But we think you need it or we wouldn't let you have it." I took some license in the use of "we."

Outside the room, I was livid, on the verge of throwing things or strangling someone. "I don't want to know who mentioned "leukemia" to Mrs. Cisneros, insensitive and inappropriate, damn it! You *never* say that to a patient or the family unless you have the evidence, the day of reckoning we'll all face in the end. What the hell is she supposed to think? Chemotherapy and a bone marrow transplant she'll never get without medical insurance? For Christ's sake, other diagnoses are in the running!"

I knew David was aghast and doubted my diagnosis. Not that he disagreed with the point at issue, feeling a bit guilty, I suspected. But he'd never seen this side of me. Patient rounds with your attending physician when you were a resident weren't supposed to be like this. Typically, the professor focused on key points and handed out pearls of wisdom, but he didn't fly off the handle. As a resident, you went on your way, looking forward to tomorrow's pearls. Today, we'd lost a bond, the bond between mentor and trainee. Or maybe it had only stretched to the breaking point. "David are with me on the need for surgery or not?"

"Yes, of course. You're the attending physician."

I heard what he said, but was he thinking "you'd better be right or you're on your own?"

The tension eased as we finished the morning. He seemed wary when he asked, "Dr. Jordan, before you go, can I tell you about a problem I'm having with one of the medical students, Barbara Engstrom?"

"You mean I have more to worry about than the team making boneheaded comments to our patients?"

I wanted to calm him, to win him back with humor. He was a great resident, a hard worker. We had three weeks to go, an eternity depending on what we had to deal with, a short marriage, a honeymoon's worth. I needed to calm myself too. "What's the problem with Barbara, David?"

"Can we talk before you discuss it with her?" He was solemn now.

"OK. Let's go to your office then."

The door closed behind us. Two chairs and a metal desk topped off the décor. The walls were bare. The office changed hands every month as the residents rotated to different wards in the hospital, no time to put the name of the current occupant on the door. I didn't get it. Why didn't the hospital give each resident a portable sign with his or her name on it when the year began to take along and put on the door at each new assignment? While we're at it, can't we put something on the walls in these damned vapid places where bad news comes down every day for patients and their families, even though the news may be conjecture and not yet definitive? Mrs. Cisneros was still in my craw, and I wasn't about to let her go.

Still, the hospital administrators didn't want to know how their "consumers" lived, suffered, or died. They were busy crunching numbers like insurance company actuaries. I know; someone has to do it, but can't we show them the reality, the consequences. Put a damn visit to the trenches on their schedule. I'll be here to guide the tour any time they deign to show up.

"So, tell me about Barbara, David."

He stiffened and sighed, feeling like a failure as I read him. Tall and lanky, mostly elbows and knees, he sat on a metal desk, folded his arms across his chest, put his feet on a chair, and looked down at me seated in the other. "Dr. Jordan, she's doing poorly on the service. She's scared of the patients and her responsibilities. I'm sure you know her medical knowledge is weak. She never has an answer to any of your questions."

"I think she's nervous, high strung, and this *is* her first crack at patient care after two years of lectures and laboratories. You think there's more to it than that?"

He went on with a heavy heart, sighing again and again. It wasn't like him. "She came to me yesterday and said she was overwhelmed, uncomfortable dealing with patients. She thinks her knowledge is inadequate, and she can't take the pressure. She wants to drop out of medical school, at least for a while."

"David, we both know you don't drop out of medical school 'for a while.' She's that upset? She doesn't seem any worse than an average third-year student starting clinical medicine. But you've worked with her more than I have."

"I've waited quite a while before bringing this up, hoping things would fall into place as she gained more confidence." He reached into the top pocket of his long white coat and pulled out a pouch of tobacco. After packing the bowl of his pipe, sighing once more, his face contorted in angst, he said. "Last night, when we were on call, she came to me in tears because she couldn't get a nasogastric tube down Mrs. Allison. It was three a.m. She'd been trying for fifteen minutes, and the patient was angry, swearing at her."

"OK, David. But that's a matter of experience. She has no confidence. Hell, we all know excellent doctors who're disasters when it comes to procedures. They have someone else to do them."

"Right, but her problem is worse than that. She doesn't understand what she wants to know when she takes a history. She doesn't know how to follow patients. The bits and pieces don't fall in place. Something's wrong with her reasoning, *what* I don't know! She won't finish the clerkship with a passing grade unless you say she has to."

"I'd never tell you that, David."

I sighed now. How could she do well enough in college to get into medical school and stumble? And she'd graduated from "boot camp," the rigorous courses of the first two preclinical years. That was a requirement for any medical student to advance to third year clinical medicine and patient care.

"Let's bring her in. Do you want to be here or should I speak to her alone?"

"She's had more than enough of me. Maybe you need some one on one time."

———

I asked Barbara to come into David's office and sit down. She was pretty, thin, and intense, fidgeting with the ear pieces on the stethoscope in her lap. Her glasses seemed to magnify the tears in her eyes. "Barbara, David just explained some of the problems you're having on the clerkship. What do think the trouble is?"

She flushed, and the tears fell freely now. Red blotches erupted on her neck. After clearing her throat a few times, she said. "I just don't feel comfortable here. My knowledge is inferior to other students, and I don't know what I'm doing or why I'm doing it half the time."

"Barbara, it was a tough transition for all of us. Every medical student feels shaky on their first clerkship, especially if it's internal medicine and your first contact with sick patients. Maybe you're being too hard on yourself."

I had an anecdote perfect for the occasion, a vignette about my own incompetence as a third-year student, though I wasn't sure I should reveal it. When I was a third year student at the Veterans Hospital in Omaha, I performed my first "circulation time" on a patient. The test determined whether shortness of breath was due to lung disease or to back up of blood in the lungs from a failing left ventricle of the heart. You put a needle into a forearm vein; the syringe holding the needle is attached to a vertical glass manometer. You let blood flow back into the manometer to measure the venous pressure which was usually elevated in heart disease but not in lung disease. Then, a bile salt solution (sodium desoxycholate) is injected forcefully into the vein after the position of the stopcock has been changed. The patient is to report the moment he tastes the bitter bile salts on his tongue. Normally, the salts would get there through the venous and arterial circulation within sixteen seconds; a longer time indicated congestion in the lung from heart failure.

I was confident I could do the test after seeing one (it was one of those procedures billed as "see one, do one, teach one."). I must have missed something in the "see one" part. When I went to inject the bile salts into the arm vein of a spry and edentulous elderly veteran, Mr. Hugh Cummings, I'd forgotten to change the position of the stopcock. Instead of going into the vein, the solution shot up the vertical manometer, hit the ceiling, and splattered down on his face. He circled and smacked his lips with his impressive tongue in his toothless state and called out with joy. "I taste it, Doc! I taste it!" Unofficially, it was the shortest 'circ' time on record, less than 0.5 seconds. And it gave new meaning to the aphorism: "The Veterans serve twice."

Barbara blurted out. "I know, but I'm inadequate! I don't like what I'm doing. I didn't think medicine would be like this. It's frightening. What if I harmed or killed a patient?"

119

I was glad I hadn't told her about Mr. Cummings. It wouldn't have helped because she was in more trouble than I realized and, she knew it. I hoped for another explanation. "Barbara, is there something else wrong, family or anything?"

"Not really, Dr. Jordan. I'm just miserable and disappointed in medical school. I don't want to go on any more, and I've never given up on anything in my life."

"Then, don't give up now! Have you talked to the Associate Dean of Students?"

"No, but I have an appointment with Dr. Williams, this afternoon."

"Good. We care, and we'll help you. Don't decide yet. Let's meet again after you've seen Dean Williams."

"OK. I promise. Thanks for you concern."

———

Dictating today's notes on the patients, I was precise on Mrs. Cisneros. I felt strongly about the diagnosis. Let's put my reputation on the line, "leukemia, my ass." The intercom buzzed while I was in mid-sentence. "Hello."

"Dean Williams' office is on the line. He wants to know if you can meet at two this afternoon. It's about one of your medical students, a Barbara Engstrom."

I hesitated. Dean Williams' day was one meeting after another. He did no patient care and no research. He was busy courting benefactors and doing damage control. Still, he decided when a meeting was held with no concern for anyone else's schedule. After all, his was full. Full of what, I didn't know. I wondered what benefit the medical school and the University Hospital gained from his scheming. "OK, tell them I'll be there."

I paged David Miller to change the time of afternoon rounds. I went back to the dictation, playing the tape again. The loud buzz on the intercom that had interrupted me was captured on the recording. "Leukemia, my ass," I'd said just before the buzz.

I erased the words; not for the transcriber to hear or type, nor, for that matter, to be seen above my name and signature in a formal note. Still, l was boiling about the point, wishing I'd said to the team. "Remember, as a physician, the dictum 'first, do no harm' also means that you never say to a patient or their family that you suspect a lethal disease until the evidence can't be ignored. Keep your suspicions to yourself, for Christ's sake. Is that clear enough?"

———

"Dean Williams can see you now, Dr. Jordan. He apologizes for keeping you waiting so long."

"Thanks, Bev."

I walked back to the Associate Dean's office through a long corridor knowing a fiasco was on tap. I'd been here before, familiar with his routine. You had the feeling you needed to count your fingers after you shook hands with Harvey Williams. He was sitting at his desk, sifting through forms when I walked in. He had weighty matters to ponder, matters the rest of us wouldn't understand. Had he thought about meeting me half way down the hall, letting go of his "power in the office" menu in a gesture of semi-sincere warmth? I would have done that. No, weighty matters were at work.

"Hi, Colin. Thanks for coming in. How are you?"

We shook hands as he stood up.

"Fine, Harvey."

All my fingers were still there. I'd never understood administrators in academic medical centers. Why would you want a job like this, so far from the stress and chaos of clinical medicine? Didn't he have "the lesion," the need to prove himself everyday caring for patients, to say nothing about the obsessive, precise, and competitive world of scientific research? His job didn't appeal to me, though I had to admit that mine had lost a bit of its sheen lately.

I took a chair as the Associate Dean sat down behind his desk. Harvey Williams was self-assured as usual. His suntan reflected off his long white coat, a tan kept alive year round by skiing trips. Why he wore a white coat at all, I had no idea. A sweat shirt and jeans would've been fine today unless dignitaries, needing to be impressed, were coming in. He smiled and leaned back in his swivel chair, cradling the back of his neck with the fingers of both hands entwined.

His diplomas and training certificates were on the wall; M.D. from Harvard Medical School, residency in internal medicine at the

Massachusetts General Hospital, and chief medical resident at Yale-New Haven Hospital; impressive for sure, his trophies, his greatest moments. He'd peaked early, and he knew how to turn it on to get where he wanted to go. He'd done nothing since. I guess he didn't have to with his pedigree. He glanced at his Rolex, and then at me from the corner of an eye, as if I were here for his bidding; in other words, a few minutes should do it.

"I understand there's a problem on your service with Barbara Engstrom. What's your take on it?"

"I just learned the extent of it this morning, Harvey. David Miller, my resident, brought it up. She's upset about her performance and feels inadequate with patients. I haven't been impressed with her so far, but I thought it was the usual third-year student jitters about starting clinical medicine and patient care. After talking to her though, it goes deeper than that. She doesn't know much about symptoms, disease, or how to deal with patients."

"Nah, sounds like typical third-year student jitters to me," he said with a smile.

"I don't think so, Harvey. How did she do in the first two years of medical school?"

The smile on Harvey Williams' face was gone. He fidgeted in his chair. He paused as if he were mulling over what his response should be. "Well, she did *pretty* well. I mean she had trouble getting through biochemistry the first year, and she barely passed pathology the second year; otherwise, no problems."

"What about Part I of the National Board Examination at the end of her second year?"

A passing score on that exam was required for advancement to the final two years of medical school, the years in which medical students began to take care of patients under supervision. The failure rate across the country on the Part I exam was about fifteen percent. Williams lit a cigarette. The pauses were getting longer.

"Colin, she failed."

"What, the biochemistry, the pathology?"

"No, all six parts."

"You mean physiology, pharmacology, microbiology, anatomy...…."

"I already said 'all six parts,' didn't I?" He had red blotches on his neck now. They were going around. Maybe it was a virus.

"Harvey, I thought the policy here was that preclinical students had to pass that exam before starting clinical training." I was beginning to sense something cryptic. I knew too that he wouldn't have told me any of this if I hadn't asked.

Williams rocketed forward in his chair and deftly placed his open palms downward on the desk. The fingers were vibrating. He riveted a gaze on me, seizing the offensive. "Colin, you obviously don't know who Barbara Engstrom is."

"No, I don't, Harvey. But I'm curious."

"She's the United Film Studios Scholar."

"What does that mean?"

"United Studios gives the medical school $7,500 each year for four years in support of a specific student. We can only give the award every four years."

"Who chooses the student?"

"Selected members of the Admissions Committee."

"The selected members made a mistake, Harvey."

Williams' hands were trembling. His sun-tanned face blanched around the eyes after a recent skiing trip. I'd seen better looking raccoons. He nearly screamed at me. "Look. We've got a hell of a problem here. Barbara Engstrom *cannot* be allowed to fail or even drop out of medical school voluntarily! Do you understand?"

There it was; no words minced. I edged forward in the chair. I knew *exactly* what I didn't like about Harvey Williams, the administrator, maybe why I'd always been suspicious of administrators isolated in their offices and committee meetings. Now, I could stop the fog from rolling in. "Wait a minute, damn it. A lot of students wouldn't mind being paid to go to medical school, would they? Imagine that; graduating with no debt. Something's wrong, Harvey. Barbara Engstrom hasn't had too bad a time of it, has she? No wonder all this hit her like a ton of bricks. She knows her only chance to graduate is to repeat the second year and try

123

to pass the National Boards. That's what every other student in her situation has had to do. You should have seen the red flags before now."

"OK, calm down! We'll set up special tutorials for her. You and Miller will work with her and get her through this clerkship."

"Oh, for Christ's sake, Harvey. Don't you see, she doesn't want that. She knows she's not cutting it. At least *she* has the sense to see that. To hell with United, they've blown a few themselves."

"You won't help us out then? Is that your stance?"

"It's not a question of helping you out. It won't work. She has surgery next. Who'll carry her through that clerkship? I don't think you'll find anyone eager to help you out in *that* department. Why don't you tell her to repeat the second year? She expects to hear it."

———

When I got back to my office, a note was on the desk.

Dear Dr. Jordan,

I wish to thank you for your concern about me. Dr. Miller and you have been very understanding. I realize now I just don't belong here. Medicine is too much for me. Maybe I'll change my mind later. In the meantime, I've applied for a secretarial position at St. Luke's Hospital in the medical records department. My knowledge of medical terminology should be an asset! I'd appreciate your writing a letter of recommendation

Thank you.

Barbara Engstrom

The note saddened me. She was naïve, even as the United Studios Scholar, whatever extra pressure that put on her. Enough stress went around just being a medical student. But you don't drop out of medical school and expect to return at your whim unless a personal or family tragedy has struck. Other qualified candidates, about whom no red flags have been raised, are lined up behind you. Didn't she realize *that* was why David and I were so upset? I called Barbara, but she didn't agree, saying she could return when it suited her, and she didn't need to repeat the second year. Maybe she knew something I didn't.

———

As I put the groceries on the shelves in my fancy walk-in pantry that evening, the phone rang. "Hi, Dr. Jordan, David Miller here."

"Hi, how's your night on call going?"

"Busy. You've got five new patients so far for tomorrow. Listen, Mrs. Cisneros just came out of the operating room. She's doing fine. The rapid tests on the abdominal lymph nodes show caseating granulomas. The acid-fast stains are positive. You were right, tuberculosis. I'm sorry I doubted your diagnosis. And I know, I shouldn't have mentioned leukemia. I guess that's why I'm the resident, and you're the attending physician."

"David, go forth and sin no more. I'll see you in the morning."

CHAPTER 9

PUS WAS ON HIS MIND

A torrent of work swept us along the next week. Patients with maladies of uncommon urgency were all over the internal medicine ward, and their diseases didn't yield to our diagnostic wisdom. Many were terribly ill, and some died. Others should have died to spare them the agony they endured, the agony we'd put them through.

When I had to call a private physician to explain how we'd failed, I had a knot in my gut. After all, the University Hospital was "Mecca," and patients were supposed to be in good hands here. I was despondent when a patient died, especially when we didn't have time to sort it out; or if we'd had time and failed, I was all the more despondent.

How do you tell someone who's not a physician what it's like to be one, what it takes every day in the foxhole, what our limitations are, and why we fail? I'll have a go at it, but I won't get it right. Many of my colleagues don't see it this way, I know, and I speak only to internal medicine where diagnosis is everything. The rest is a lot easier.

We have truths, but not as many as we need. Some problems are clear. By 1977, we knew from elegant studies by the Veterans Administration and others in Framingham, Massachusetts that hypertension was by far the most common cause of congestive heart failure and stroke. Treatment of hypertension was essential to prevent those complications. Before then, coronary artery and valvular heart disease were thought to cause nearly all cases of congestive heart failure.

We know what the best antibiotic therapy is for certain infections – meningitis, pneumonia, sepsis (blood poisoning), urinary tract infections,

127

gangrene and so on, at least until the next resistant organism shows up. But *what* causes rheumatoid arthritis, systemic lupus, leukemia, lymphoma or ulcerative colitis? We haven't a clue. Of course, I think they're all caused by viruses. We just haven't caught the culprit red-handed.

In a hundred years, maybe twenty, our future colleagues will laugh at our ignorance just as we laugh now at the medicine of yesteryear. We go on. What I don't like is pretending we know more than we do. What we need to say is that medicine is murky with plenty of guess work to go with the science. At times, the question comes down to: How precise is your guess work?

We know more about treatment than we do about how diseases work and what causes them despite decades of research; the diseases are smarter and tougher then we are. "Treatment guidelines" and algorithms sprang up for many diseases in 1977. Some of it had to do with pharmaceutical companies developing new products and pushing them; again, the focus was on treatment. From press reports and television programs, you'd think we always know what's going on; true maybe seventy percent of the time.

But things get murkier when a physician doesn't have a diagnosis. No substitute there, a diagnosis is everything. You can use all the treatment guidelines you want, but they don't work if you don't have the diagnosis right. And often, the diseases don't behave the way the textbooks say they do. It's particularly hard for University Hospital physicians who aren't usually there at the beginning of a patient's illness; most patients are referred after no one else had been able to figure out what's going on. By then, the waters are muddied by biases that haven't held up and by treatments that have broken down or done harm.

What is it then that makes an exceptional physician, one who's wrong a little less often than the rest? Most likely, it's humility, a willingness to admit that you don't know what's going on. Once you get that out of the way, you're free to create, to plumb your depths when you tackle the unknown and the unknowable.

Of course, medical knowledge is crucial. For sure, there's no short cut when it comes to that. Important also is judgment which is harder to define. Sometimes it shows when a physician blows off goofy test results that don't make sense. Or he or she is willing to take risks that may mean doing nothing until the smoke clears. Sometimes you need to get out of the way and let patients heal themselves on a short leash in case they do the patient harm. Or it may mean taking unconventional and aggressive risk, a lonely undertaking. You'd better have a good idea what you're doing or at least a working hypothesis.

You might think experience is crucial. I don't know now after more than thirty-five years in medicine as I write. Sure it is for a surgeon. You don't want a novice trying to replace the aortic valve in your heart or repairing a ruptured aneurysm in your brain.

But internal medicine and diagnostic work are different. Failure to make a diagnosis is every internist's nightmare. Physicians who are exceptional now were exceptional from square one, during their training. And, as residents, we knew who they were. Instinct and savvy trumps experience every time. If experience is gained without skepticism and critical examination, it doesn't add to a physician's skill; it dulls it. If you've seen it all before, you deal with it as you always have. Then the diagnosis bites you when it's not what you thought.

An exceptional physician agonizes more over defeat than he or she celebrates victory, and you'll have plenty of defeats to go with a handful of triumphs. The patient needs a special physician when the diagnosis is on the line, someone comfortable flying by the seat of their pants, armed to the teeth with fundamentals - knowledge, judgment, skepticism and courage – and yes, experience looked at over and again. And then, throw in the guts and doggedness of a long distance runner.

Maybe that's why they say we "practice" medicine. You usually don't get it quite right as if you're learning to play an instrument. After a while, that's OK. You know you never will.

————

David Miller was a more humble and astute physician every day. He was in his stretch run, ready to start a distinguished career as a primary care general internist in private practice. The carnage around us humbled me too, but I didn't see anything we'd missed or done wrong. The mutual torment that bred respect and camaraderie drew us closer. We didn't hear about Barbara Engstrom again. I was surprised that Harvey Williams and the administration had given up.

A week after the Engstrom episode, Paul Webb, another medical student on our inpatient service, was brought to the Emergency Room by his girlfriend at one in the morning. He had fever and couldn't speak; he had no movement in his right arm or leg. David evaluated him with precision and dispatch. While the intern was doing a spinal tap, he rushed to make a call from his office.

I rolled over in bed, trying to find the ringing menace. I didn't respond to this kind of abuse the way I'd done as a resident; nor did I wake up with the same clarity. Now, fear filled my humbled heart, that fear of knowing how easily it could all go wrong and slip away. Maybe it was because I was now the physician responsible for what happened to the patients or, for that matter, to the medical students.

"Dr. Jordan, I'm sorry to wake you. David Miller here. One of your third-year students, Paul Webb, was just admitted to the ward. He's been sick three or four days with headache and left-sided facial pain. He didn't say anything to me about it. Earlier tonight, he developed fever and couldn't speak to his girlfriend on the phone. On exam, he has a temperature of 103 degrees and a right-sided paralysis with expressive aphasia."

Expressive aphasia is the clinical term for a state in which a person can't say what they mean, even though they know what they want to say; it comes out all wrong. It's usually caused by a lesion near or compressing on the speech center in the brain.

"We did a spinal tap. They're just handing me the results. It shows 200 cells, all lymphocytes. That's all I know. I'm worried about herpes simplex virus encephalitis."

"David, order sinus films and a CAT scan. Herpes encephalitis is a good thought, but it could be an abscess in his brain or a subdural empyema."

"Can you hurry in? I'm scared. I wish they'd sent him to another service. He's on station 8-C, by the way."

"I'll be there in twenty minutes."

Driving in, I focused on Webb, feeling a bit guilty. I hadn't paid him much attention; he hadn't needed any. He wasn't a big kid, but he was an ox at five-foot-nine and around a hundred-and-eighty pounds. Brilliant, mature, and humble, his blond hair was crew cut, and his green eyes darted back and forth, nervous on his first case presentations. You knew he'd be a leader in medicine and in life. Tonight, he'd have our attention and steal our hearts.

When I got there, his parents were waiting. His mother wept quietly as I introduced myself and left to examine him. I may have been a bit abrupt, but I was eager to see him, to get to the bottom of it. I didn't like to talk when I wasn't ready.

David was right to suspect encephalitis due to herpes simplex virus which caused a unique form of the disease involving only a portion of one side of the brain, but it wouldn't have explained the facial pain. The x-rays showed inflammation with a large collection of fluid in his sinuses. The CAT scan was ambiguous. I was concerned about a collection of pus under pressure above one side of his brain ("subdural empyema").

We called in a neurosurgeon. An ear, nose and throat surgeon was also summoned and took Webb to surgery for drainage of his paranasal sinuses. She removed a large amount of pus with some improvement in the paralysis and speech difficulties. The procedure told us that he had a connection between the sinuses and the meninges (the lining membranes of the brain), probably due to a breakdown in normal anatomic barriers.

I discussed it with the neurosurgeon, John Bolger. "John, I think he has a subdural empyema in spite of the equivocal CAT scan. We've started him on antibiotics, but if the neurological signs come back, he'll need a carotid artery angiogram to make the diagnosis."

"I'm not so sure. The new computerized scans are highly accurate in my experience and much less risky than angiography. Let's just sit tight and see what happens."

"But I don't think CAT scans have been studied enough for detection of a pus collection over one side of the brain. I don't trust them. I agree they're excellent when there's an abscess in the brain tissue."

I hadn't realized how suspicious I was of new technology even though I was less than four years out of training. Enthusiasm surged when new tests came out because we wanted to be rid of riskier procedures that needed highly skilled specialists. Eventually Bolger would be right; more advanced CAT scans would replace angiography, just not tonight.

I went to Paul's room after the sinus procedure. I hadn't had a chance to examine him. He was waking up from the anesthetic. Mr. and Mrs. Webb sat at the bedside holding hands; Mr. Webb sobbed quietly, listing his forehead on the left side of his wife's shoulder and neck, much as Molly McGinnis at Harborview had done on mine, bless her.

"Paul, squeeze my fingers as hard as you can. You know the drill from the physical diagnosis course." He'd been a student of mine in the course a year ago. I inserted my second and third fingers into each of his hands. I'd forgotten he'd been a student gymnast. I shouldn't have said "as hard as you can;" we always say that to patients. He took me literally as he was supposed to and crushed my fingers. I winced and nearly yelped in pain, though I welcomed the power in his grip. He turned to me. "Dr. Jordan, it was expressive aphasia."

Behind the bandages, the rascal's eyes twinkled as if he had me over a barrel which he didn't. In a sense, he was Paul the Vietnam veteran I'd run into at the laundry though this Paul's eyes sent another signal. Still, a vulnerable son was in trouble again, and I was here. Was there a difference? Did I care more for Paul Webb because he was a medical student and not a derelict? I shouldn't by my calling, and I didn't think so.

Still, the scene had something to it I couldn't quite put my newly crushed finger on. I had to admit he was the best medical student I'd known. He was a hell of lot smarter and a hell of a lot more composed than I was at his age, and an All-America gymnast to boot. I couldn't handle my emotion and felt faint as I looked at his parents, hoping not to give myself away. I thought about the Paul lying in his vomit at the laundry, the Paul whose parents I hadn't met as I dug in to deal with the son I had in front of me.

"Yeah, I know, Paul. That's right. But leave the diagnostic work to David and me tonight, okay? We'll present your case later at a conference when you can comment on the proceedings!"

My heart had been moved by many a patient in my young career. But here, I was dealing with a *melange* of courage and knowledge with courage ever the more important, yet a patient who knew enough to imagine pus pressing on his brain or a malignant tumor infiltrating his will. He was mulling over his diagnosis, and it didn't look good. That's how he was different from Paul, the Vietnam veteran. And tonight, he was my son in his vulnerable and knowing state. He was everyone's son and a brilliant one at that. His star shone bright if he had a future, if we could keep him one. If God grants us His grace, Paul Webb will not die or end up "brain dead" on my watch tonight.

Hours later, his paralysis and speech defects came back. I insisted on an angiogram, nearly having another tantrum in front of David Miller. Within the hour, a physician in the radiology suite injected contrast dye directly into the left carotid artery of Paul's neck. Wearing masks and surgical gowns, David and I stood in solidarity next to the radiologist. Paul was sedated. Within seconds of the injection, a crop of hives erupted over the left side of his face, an accelerated allergic reaction to the contrast material, potentially life-threatening anaphylaxis.

"Oh, hell!" The radiologist said. "Shit! He's allergic to the dye. Don't anyone panic! Let's give him some epinephrine (adrenalin) right now, stat."

"I agree, Ben," I butted in. "Now we're here, let's get what we need."

We had the films in half-an-hour. A large opaque mass compressed the left side of Paul's brain, suggesting a collection of pus or fluid above; no abscess in the brain. The allergic reaction had subsided after two doses of epinephrine, and he was stable.

We called John Bolger, and he agreed with the diagnosis. While I explained the problem to Paul's parents, the nurses shaved his head urgently for surgery. David Miller had the evening off after spending the previous day and night in the hospital, but he wanted to stay until the outcome was clear. "I won't be able to sleep anyway."

During the surgery, we reviewed other patients, talked about Barbara Engstrom, and discussed David's career plans. The main goal was to keep each other awake. About 6:30 a.m., a page said that Paul was in the recovery room. David and I dashed several flights down the stairwell. When we got there, Bolger was writing his postoperative orders at the nursing station.

"Well, what did you find?" David blurted out.

"A hundred milliliters of pus over the left cerebral hemisphere. God, it was putrid, smelled awful! Everything went fine. We repaired a defect in a membrane, the dura behind the maxillary sinus; a leak there was the source of the trouble."

"Oh, thank God!" I collapsed in a chair next to Bolger. "We'll go to the lab and look at the stains of the pus. If antibiotics need changing, we'll write the orders. Thanks, John. You were magnificent."

Was he ever! We had a son at our bosom now. I couldn't wait to see his parents. I was strange and giddy, a giddiness that sometimes comes on me after terror and heartache. The "all clear" signal had gone off again as it had after the bombing I'd known as a kid in England.

After we'd looked at the lab stains, David and I went back to recovery to examine Paul and alter the antibiotic therapy. I was exhausted, fading into coma with a headache. I laid my head in my arms folded on a counter at the nursing station. We must have dozed off. I thought I'd said to David, "I love that kid, and I love you too," but maybe I'd only dreamt it. "You're a hell of a resident. You should go into infectious diseases."

I loved everyone at that moment. Now, can someone tell me about the Vietnam veteran at the laundry? Had he stuck with it at the Wadsworth VA? David, who was more exhausted than me, asked: "Did you say something, Dr. Jordan?"

I didn't know what I'd said, but I didn't retract it. "David, take the morning off. I'll handle the patients with the intern until you get in." He'd been at the top of his class at Michigan. It must be a hell of a medical school. Rounds were an hour away. But he was here at 7:30 as usual. Harry, the intern and I made rounds, but they weren't routine. Neither Barbara Engstrom nor Paul Webb was here to fill us in on their patients. We did our best, but we weren't efficient.

––––––

I'm not heady now after being right. Blunders get your attention more than triumphs ever do. Now that you know about Paul Webb, I want to tell you about Clarence Struthers, a patient in my keep for a night when I was a junior resident at the Seattle VA. He's never left me, a gentle fifty-five-year-old black man with a purple heart for bravery in the segregated armed forces of World War II. The resident in charge summarized his case before she went home for the night. My job was to make sure that Clarence was in his room in the morning and not in the morgue.

"A piece of cake," I thought. After all, the tough sledding had been done. With coronary artery disease and a history of heart attacks, he was here after six fainting spells within twenty-four hours. He was in complete heart block, a condition in which the natural sinus pacemaker of the heart loses track of the ventricles to which it tries to send impulses. His heart rate (pulse) was eighteen beats a minute when he was admitted, a heart rate that wouldn't keep him awake or upright for long. Ole Olson at Harborview had had the same problem.

That day, Clarence had a permanent mechanical pacemaker put in. They were new, and we didn't know much about them. The evening he was on my watch, the nurse said he wanted to talk. "Doc, I have a funny feeling tonight. I can't quite explain it, but I think I'm going to die."

When a patient says that, the doctor pays attention because the patient might be right. I did. "Mr. Struthers, you're out of the woods now. If you were going to die, you'd have died yesterday. Now, the pacemaker will keep you going. You're in great shape."

His eyes brightened and a big smile crossed his face. He reached out to shake my hand. "OK, Doc. Thanks for listening. I guess I'm just scared. You're very kind."

"No, not at all, Clarence. I'm honored to be involved in your care."

I walked twenty feet across the hall to finish dictating. Less than two minute later, an alarm went off, and he had a cardiac arrest. We couldn't revive him. I didn't know what had happened. The cardiac monitor showed that the pacemaker was still firing.

I quietly sobbed myself to sleep in the residents' quarters, trying not to wake anyone up. I was the last person Clarence had smiled at or shaken hands with. It wasn't so much that I could have done more for him except maybe temper my naïve and, as it turned out, false assurances.

I'd never before, nor have I since, learned so much from an autopsy. Clarence had had so many coronaries that his heart didn't have enough living muscle to respond to the electrical impulses of the pacemaker. The miracle machine was stimulating unresponsive scar tissue. The pacemaker hadn't failed; his heart couldn't respond. In fact, the tip of the electrode had perforated his non-existent heart muscle and was protruding into his chest cavity, firing into thin air. I had no idea this could happen. I wasn't consoled when his case was discussed at a "mortality conference," and no one else did either.

That was the problem with the latest devices and procedures; they promised us everything, "a new dawn" as advertisements said in medical journals, but it took us years to sort out the truth. Still, I was in charge that night, and I'd told Mr. Struthers in my "doctor's voice" that he was "out of the woods" and "in good shape." I was disconsolate for weeks.

Medicine has no room for arrogance, ignorance, or false confidence. I don't know how many times I've thought of Clarence in his last moments. Today, he'd get a heart transplant paid for by the Veterans Administration. Life is precious and in constant danger of being lost, especially if you live in an era before the real miracles and new dawns are here.

CHAPTER 10

A THREE-LEGGED STOOL

I'd been at the University Hospital four years now. On a morning in spring, I got a call from the secretary in the Division of Infectious Diseases. She said I needed to make an appointment to see Dr. William L. Hewitt. I knew something was up because Bill and I had lunch often, and he'd never asked me to make an appointment.

Bill was my boss, in his mid-sixties, winding down. He was chief of the Division of Infectious Diseases in the Department on Internal Medicine. When he wasn't in clinic or on the infectious diseases consultation service, he worked at home in Malibu. With his status, he no longer had to cover the internal medicine ward. At first pass, he was a *bon vivant*. You could dismiss him as a light weight from an academic standpoint, but you'd be wrong. Many of his patients were movie stars, entertainers, politicians, or well-known business entrepreneurs as you might expect at the University Hospital in Los Angeles. He was also a gifted physician I revered.

"Colin, I just got the results of your fourth-year appraisal from the promotions committee. It's a preliminary projection of your chances of reaching tenure at the level of associate professor."

I was all ears.

He wore a short-sleeved shirt and a bow tie as usual. I'd always liked his even and easy keel. Bill had worked hard to recruit me to the University Hospital four years ago. He was the boss I wanted. He'd left me alone, trusting me, content to see what sort of research I'd come up with in

Dr. Steven Jackson's laboratory. Now, I was about to find out how well it had worked.

"You know, an assistant professor here has seven years to reach associate professor or have his or her appointment terminated. Your teaching and clinical evaluations are superb, Colin, maybe the best in the Department of Internal Medicine. The house staff and students can't say enough about you. And your presentations at conferences have been models for the department. The Dean, Dr. Sherman, goes around saying that you're 'the doctor's doctor.' You know this, I'm sure. I don't mean to minimize it, probably enough to get you promoted to associate professor."

I knew what was coming. He hadn't said a word about "research," and he was going to. He went about it in the way I'd have done if I were him. First, give the positives and then bring up the problems. "When I recruited you, I thought you were one of those rare people who'd be a top flight scientist as well as an outstanding physician and teacher. I still do. You have the tools. I know you're having problems. Christ, I went through a nasty divorce twenty years ago, and I remember what it was like. I still have oozing sores and scars all over my soul like some sort of parasitic infestation."

He leaned back in his swiveled chair and smiled at me. He'd amused himself. A chuckle escaped his throat and reverberated around the office as he tilted his head back and winked. As if he were now immune to havoc, his past was full of harmless and humorous reminiscences. As best I could tell, Bill had always survived his traumas through humor. Now, he seemed to be saying "don't take all this too seriously." I smiled back though I didn't believe for a moment that I'd ever remember it with a knowing chuckle. He was serious again now.

"You were highly productive at the CDC, but not as much here. In a place like this, the name of the game is 'what have you done lately?' I know you have good research going, excellent findings on the herpes viruses. You need to publish your work and apply for your own grants. You have to get out from under Steven Jackson's wing and strike out on your own. I'm not far from retirement. I need to think about a successor now. I'd like to turn this job over to you, but it's not entirely up to me. To make that possible, you *have* to get going on the research. Otherwise, they'll bring in an outsider. You know, new blood with no baggage and no loyalty to the old regime."

As the most junior member in the division of infectious diseases, I mumbled something I hoped sounded like appreciation. To take on his challenge, I'd need to muster a commitment to my research that had eluded me. A few years ago, it was clear-cut. I had the aspirations he'd described. That's why I was at the University Hospital. Now, other matters gripped and confused me.

———

In the evening, restless and agitated, I careened around the apartment. Bill Hewitt was on my mind. It was scorching hot for some reason in April, and pungent smog had moved in too soon in the year. Even inside the apartment, my eyes were burning.

A traffic jam on Wilshire Boulevard had drivers in frenzy, horns honking like an orchestra warming up to play Bartok or Janacek out of tune. I walked down Wellesley Avenue to the corner at Wilshire and still couldn't figure out what was wrong; three lanes of cars were backed up, heading east to Westwood. I walked as far as the "Bicycle Shop Café," where I often took residents and medical students to dinner after a month on service.

An agitated fellow, tall and slender, leaned up against an overheated car stuck in the middle lane on Wilshire. His hair struck me first; it was greasy black and styled in a "duck tail," then, the tattoos. He was a character called "Vinnie" or "Vito" I'd seen in snippets of a television program. He yelled at me about a fire in a canyon near Bel Air and another one in Topanga Canyon. Sirens screamed in the distance. Because the canyons were about twelve miles apart, I wondered if the fires had been set. In Southern California, we always worried about that, more so when the Santa Ana winds blew in the fall.

"Can you believe this shit, Man?" He bellowed. "And it's my fuckin' anniversary! Great huh?"

"She'll understand when she hears about it," I yelled back. "Just don't talk to her like that."

"Ya wanna have a beer togetha in that restaurant behind you? I have time now, goin' fuckin' nowhere."

"No, I don't think so. Hang in there. I have to go. Happy anniversary!"

I'd been a pompous ass. What the hell did I know about how he spoke to his wife? Maybe she liked him talking to her like that, and maybe she gave it back in kind. It may have had something to do with Bill Hewitt. Or maybe it was the New Jersey accent, the East Coast "in your face" attitude that made me cringe. When I was growing up in Garden Grove, a family from New Jersey moved in next door to us in the duplex. We never had a quiet moment or the slightest uncertainty about anything after they got there. Maybe it was none of that but something stuck in my craw tonight.

I thought of my office as a way to escape the smog and the din, but the traffic jam kept me home. Stewing in the apartment, I felt dishonest for not telling Bill Hewitt I didn't know where I stood.

If you hoped to reach a pinnacle in academic medicine, to be a division chief or a department chair, you had to sit on "a three-legged stool." The first leg was patient care where excellence was expected. The second was teaching, excellence a given there too. The third leg, research, had most of the junior faculty stampeding for the exits to go into private practice after they'd put in five or six years hoping against hope for promotion and tenure. Bill Hewitt didn't want that for me. We were all pawns in a treacherous game.

The survivors on the stools showed their mettle by bringing in big money from the National Institutes of Health, the NIH. That was the currency that counted. Never mind that two legs of the stool were creaking and wobbling now as "the superstars" spent more time on research and on NIH committees than they did on patient care or teaching. The University didn't care as long as money and prestige flowed in as it sent out press releases announcing the latest grants.

When a scientist won an award, the University got an additional forty-eight percent of the total in indirect costs or overhead, often several hundred thousand dollars per award. You can imagine the amount of money involved if a hundred professors were bringing in grants. The University made it plenty clear which leg on the stool wasn't allowed to wobble. Later on though, the medical residents cringed when they learned that the next attending physician on their ward full of patients with no diagnosis was a research superstar, recently profiled in the Los Angeles Times. They often had a hidden "back-up attending" they could call for advice on their sickest patients.

I'd done well in research training. Now, the goals of that time were vague and remote; far easier to be a naive trainee full of ideas who had a mentor raising money to keep the laboratory afloat. So, the salary of a critical technician or research associate was secure for a couple of years. But then what? I knew what; more proposals for funding, endless hours to prepare with no assurance that they'd be reviewed fairly. The men in charge of funding committees at the NIH had your fate in their hands, committed to their beliefs, infatuated with the latest "novel concept" that might be forgotten or spurned altogether next year. And, of course, the "prestigious" laboratories took home most of the bacon. Some others misrepresented or even fabricated data and took home bits of bacon too.

The "turn around time" for a proposal to be funded or rejected was nine months. The success rate for first applications hovered around eight percent. How was a scientist to plan for recruitment and retention of staff members? And, on top of that, as a physician competing with Ph.D. scientists, you had to know your field in patient care as well as you knew basic science, both of which were constantly changing. And there was no overlap between them. Ph.D. scientists concentrated solely on their research and gave a few lectures to the graduate students. As a physician with demanding patient care duties, you'd come out ahead in this game?

The elation I'd felt with each success didn't do much for me now. After a research paper was published, I was pressed to come up with another. Was there something wrong with being a good doctor and teacher, accepting with grace the rewards due you? What was this high-minded notion to be at the forefront of medicine to give new knowledge to your colleagues they didn't know they needed? How arrogant and presumptuous it seemed, and how thinly it wore now. I had the towel in my hand, ready to throw it in the ring to stop the fight. Call in the "fight doctor." He'd know what to do.

"Let the committees have their shitty little piece of the world, the arrogant bastards," I thought. "What does it matter? Give it to them. Let them salivate about how to screw over the next application from a young assistant professor trying to start his or her career. Let them shove the next 'novel concept' you-know-where."

I'd give Bill Hewitt a decision in the morning or maybe the day after tomorrow. I wasn't comfortable on the three-legged stool tonight. The traffic jam was still on a half block away. A shoving match had started when I walked back to Wilshire. I wrote off the night and read "The Bell Jar" by Sylvia Plath. I still had a lot to learn about me or anyone who wanted to tell a story.

CHAPTER 11

THE EMMA LAZARUS CLINIC

I held an infectious diseases clinic on Tuesday and Friday morning. The clinic was inefficient, chaotic, and insane. Nothing went right, and you never knew what was next. On this Tuesday, here I was again.

When I looked at it objectively, the clinic seemed professional enough with examining rooms jutting off a long corridor. Nurses wore uniforms then and spruced up spirits. I worried that our clinic couldn't compete with others that catered to the "Stars." Still, with our patients, land mines were sure to go off. You just didn't know which ones or when. Compared to inpatient medicine, the patients were, of course, not as sick. Some weren't sick at all, and others didn't want to "get better."

"The clinic of last resort" was where doctors sent patients they couldn't sort out, whether or not an infection was likely or even remotely possible. I guess they worried that pus might be festering in a recess somewhere in the body on their examining table. Eventually, they threw hands up in frustration; time for a referral to the infectious diseases specialist. Those guys thrive on obscurity and perversity.

In a dumping ground, I did my best to stop the buck, but I lost more rounds than I won. On a minor scale, it came down to a couple of lines in "The Colossus," the poem Emma Lazarus wrote for the Statue of Liberty. "Give me your tired, your poor, your huddled masses yearning to breath free, the wretched refuse of your teeming shore." But here, the poem read. "Give me your miseries, your mysteries, the unknowable and the deviant, whether sick or not, especially if they have no health insurance. Get back to me as soon as you can or take over the case if you want."

143

To do them proud, my specialties of internal medicine and infectious diseases demanded a thorough review of symptoms, details about exposure to animals, travel, mosquito and tick bites, hiking and camping, painstaking reviews of medical records and temperature curves. An infectious diseases specialist had attention to detail to give his patients and his colleagues. That was it. And it took time, a lot of time. The doggedness and the breadth of knowledge needed to do it well didn't appeal to most physicians.

We didn't perform cardiac catheterizations or bronchial endoscopies or make a lot of money. In fact, I'd never felt like a real sub-specialist. I was an internist plying the hobby I loved, infectious diseases, about half the time. The rest of the time, I was an internist and damned proud of it.

I got away with it because they came up with the first infectious diseases board examination in 1972; it was given every other year. I finished my training in 1973 and took the exam in 1974 with seven other candidates sitting in student desks in a classroom. Over six hundred doctors took the cardiology exam across the way in a sloping auditorium. For our intimate infectious diseases exam, the proctor called out the name of each candidate before he or she came forward to pick up the test materials. Our torment had a quaint feel to it.

Three of the candidates were giants in the field who'd written the scientific papers and the textbook we'd all read to take the exam. The rest of us were just us. I worried about our chances of outdoing the giants. You found out how you did by the thickness of the envelope you got in the mail a few months later. If it was thin, you had a two line congratulatory note. If it was thick, you had the application for the next test, two years hence. To this day, I have no idea who passed, but I had a thin envelope. Rumor had it that at least one of the giants had gotten a thick one. Maybe his expertise was too narrowly focused.

From a business standpoint, my practice gave nightmares to the financial managers in the Department of Internal Medicine. One had recently said to me. "Infectious diseases, it's a subspecialty we have to offer, I guess for education of residents and students, but it sure doesn't do much financially for us."

But then, I'd chosen my path years ago after reading a novel, "The Citadel" by A. J, Cronin. In it, the brilliant Scottish writer spoke of the tribulations and rare victories of a family physician caring for workers in a mining town in Wales. I'd wanted to be him, a "generalist" rather than a narrowly focused specialist. At times, I wondered how wisely I'd chosen. What was wrong with ear, nose, and throat or dermatology except that the latter was a rather superficial specialty?

This Tuesday morning, the first patient was Linda Lesser, a young folk singer whose star was shooting up in the heavens. The nurse who'd put her into the examining room had seen her give a scintillating performance two weeks ago at "The Troubadour" in Hollywood and was excited to meet her.

Linda had been referred to the "Joint and Rheumatic Diseases Center" at the University by her private physician. For months, she'd complained of worsening muscle aches all over her body. Her physical examinations were normal, and the muscles were not tender. None of her diagnostic blood work showed elevated markers of inflammation, such as the erythrocyte sedimentation rate or the C-reactive protein. If she had enough inflammation of her muscles ("myositis") to account for the symptoms, those tests and others should have been elevated.

Nonetheless, she'd undergone two surgical muscle biopsies, and nothing had been found. Now, she was referred to me to "rule out an occult infection" before starting therapy with immune-suppressing medications to treat a collagen-vascular disease called "polymyositis." The treatment would be dangerous if there were an underlying infection. Something didn't add up.

I was annoyed when physicians, who couldn't explain "mysterious" symptoms, blamed *"a cryptic infectious process of some sort."* Their dictations often used that phrase, saying in effect, "I have no idea what's wrong with this patient." Fair enough, but they had no idea what the "infection" might be either, as if they'd never taken a course in microbiology or given it any thought. Maybe that was our sliver of leverage in infectious diseases, to take advantage of a lack of confidence about viruses, parasites, fungi, bacteria, or anything else doctors couldn't see with the naked eye or probe with a scope. Between microbes and men, that's where the final battle is so often fought, and there it's so often won or lost. In general though, we weren't a greedy lot, and I didn't see us reaping a harvest in spite of financial managers pushing for more revenue.

What other explanation was there? "It has to be an infection, doesn't it?" Yeah, but maybe an "infection" caused by the "schizococcus" I'd

145

come to realize. None of this had been brought up by the professors when I was in medical school. You were on your own in this wasteland.

Before going into Linda's room, I read the history as a twist on the "VIP" syndrome where a celebrity is referred to narrowly-focused specialists who want to help and order too many tests. All too often, they ignore or misinterpret data looking for a solution they think lies within the realm of "sophisticated" medical testing. But no medical test, no matter how good the positive or negative predictive value, will detect an illness that has an emotional basis. At some point, the "seat of the pants" has to kick in. That's the job of a primary care physician who knows the patient best. We all need a primary care physician to fight for us, to stand firm, and to insist that testing be stopped to deal with the real issue. It's the toughest job in medicine and the least appreciated by patients and families who've been conditioned to believe that they need a specialist for any organ that might go awry. The situation is aggravated when a patient is referred to Mecca with "a complex and obscure illness."

Linda was charming and depressed. Her husband answered every question I asked during the history. I tried to give him an excuse to leave the room but he didn't take hints. Just as I was on the verge of insisting that he leave, his pager went off. After a few sighs and exasperated gestures, he bolted like a bull busting through fences to get to a phone.

Now, Linda's story changed, and she told me without saying so that she lived in an emotional vacuum. She was stifled in her career and in her marriage. All the signs of depression were there; she woke up every morning at 5 a.m. with lower back pain, unable to go back to sleep. She felt isolated and useless. The muscle aches were severe, and she "had no energy." She cried a lot "for no reason" when she was alone. She wasn't interested in "life or the world." Only when singing could she feel emotion or express it, "mostly in sad songs," she said, allowing herself a wry smile.

As she spoke, the look on her face and her distant stare told me the story. She was tortured, courageous, and resolute. She was troubled and saddened by an aspect of her life. Did she know what it was? I couldn't tell. Would we get to it in this appointment, I didn't know. I did know her pain was deep, palpable, and unrelenting.

After my examination, which was completely normal, she asked. "So, do you think it's only in my head, Doctor?"

I was surprised at the question. I'd assumed she thought she had a mysterious disease, needing the kind of scrutiny only Mecca could provide. But she had inkling, maybe even hope, that it wasn't so. "I wouldn't put it that way, Linda. I don't like that expression. It's the word "only" I don't like. If it's in your mind, your body hears about it sooner or later and vice-versa. The mind and the body sometimes get out of "synch." We don't know all we need to about it. But you don't have polymyositis. That's the good news. You'll be fine if we can…

Her husband burst in, clutching his pager. Frustrated with the interruption, I was steadfast, stubborn yet again. I wanted to talk about depression. When I brought it up, he interrupted. "No! She has polymyositis, inflammation in her muscles. It's one of the collagen-vascular diseases in case you don't know about it, Doctor! I've looked into it in detail. It's not an infection. I don't know why we're seeing you anyway. Let me put it bluntly. I'm a producer in the film business, and I'm busy. I like to 'seal the deal.' Do you know what that means, Doctor? What will it take to do that with you to give her the therapy she so desperately needs?"

I knew a lot about polymyositis, a disease related to lupus (systemic lupus erythematosis or SLE), one of a group of collagen-vascular diseases. The infectious diseases specialist had to know those diseases as well as he knew malaria or histoplasmosis because the symptoms, particularly at the outset, often mimicked infection. I didn't know much about film producers, but I was learning. After resisting an impulse to say "you're an obnoxious jackass from a galaxy I know nothing about and don't care to," I said, "I'm sorry, Neil. It doesn't add up. The muscle enzymes and the two biopsies were normal which excludes that diagnosis. I want to prevent treatment with immunosuppressive drugs that could be harmful."

"Well, this is a hell of a runaround, isn't it? First, we're told that she has polymyositis, and we come to see you, an infectious diseases specialist of all things. Then, with no training in psychiatry, you say that it's depression which is ridiculous. She hasn't been depressed a day in her life, have you, Honey?" She shook her head "no," looking forlorn. Her eyes moistened.

I knew that a diagnosis of depression wouldn't set well with Neil. Of course, Linda had "never been depressed a day in her life." To him, the term meant that she'd "caused her own problems" and was, therefore, a "defective person," who couldn't "just pull herself together." Or maybe it meant he was the problem. He wouldn't understand how difficult it was for a person depressed "to seal the deal." I marveled at the courage and determination of a young woman who'd given a masterful performance at The Troubadour despite a toxic milieu of marital and medical misogyny.

"OK, Linda and Neil, we've got work to do. I'm referring Linda for psychological counseling, possibly psychotherapy, or even medical treatment for depression, if necessary. Here are the business cards of two people I recommend. They're good human beings. Keep in touch, and let me know how it goes. I'll update the Joint and Rheumatic Diseases Center on my recommendations."

As they were leaving, Neil had another page. I said to her. "It's vital for you. Please call one of these doctors, Linda. Ask them to call me for more information." I gave her my card. She nodded, gave me a kiss on the cheek, and said, "Thank you so much, Doctor. I think I know what I need to do."

———

Looking back on it, as much as I'd disliked Neil, not everything he'd said was lost on me. Was it presumptuous or arrogant to make a diagnosis of depression when I wasn't trained in psychiatry, after more experienced physicians had come to a different conclusion? Maybe I was the jackass from another galaxy.

As an internist, rather than an infectious diseases specialist, I didn't think so. In fact, an internist has to protect patients from narrowly focused specialists, protect them from their spouses, and, most of all, from themselves. After reviewing the evidence in the history, the physical examinations, and the laboratory data, and drawing on experience, an internist with an open mind has to trust his or her instincts no matter what the sub-specialists think.

But the prospect of being wrong, missing a diagnosis that was the cause of the patient's symptoms, sometimes held the internist back. Therein lay the conundrum of reliance on training, experience and instincts. Often it led to an isolated, unpopular, and risky stance. Nonetheless, I felt that more harm than good had been done by physicians unwilling to accept or tolerate that risk, who then recommended endless rounds of testing and referrals, often at the insistence of the patient or the family, doctors who wilted under pressure.

All this, of course, put off squaring up to the real problem. Depression, the mystery illness we don't understand and no one wants as a diagnosis with its profusion of symptoms; a disease where the patient, summoning courage and wrestling with brutal self-criticism, takes the reigns to heal herself with the help of a physician. And the physician had better be ready for blood all over the premises.

———

The next patient was Paul Webb, the medical student who was on my inpatient service when pus under pressure compressed half his brain. I was surprised to see him so soon. He'd just been discharged. He was my delight today in a clinic full of acrimony and aggravation. "So, how are you, young man?"

"I feel much better, Dr. Jordan. I have complete function of the right side of my body, and my speech is back to normal."

"You were very sick, Paul. You had me worried. I hope it didn't show. Let's have a look at you." I examined him in detail. Remarkably, the strength in his right arm and leg was normal though I didn't make the mistake again of asking him to squeeze my fingers as hard as he could. Subtle and sensitive tests of his ability to speak and comprehend were normal too. I removed his bandages to see a diagonal scar extending from a point behind his left ear to the midpoint of his left eyebrow. It was healing nicely. "You're doing well. Everything looks great."

"You know, Dr. Jordan, this whole thing got me to thinking. When I started on the service with you, I was impressed by how much medicine you knew, especially outside infectious diseases. But when you were taking care of me, you were on another level. I know there were disagreements about how my case should've been handled. But I also knew you'd settle for nothing less than the right course, no matter who got upset. I'm going to train in infectious diseases and go into academic medicine."

"It was a team effort, Paul. You know I often say 'these surgeons can be a pain in the ass but, when you need one, you need a damned good one.' You had a great one in John Bolger, bless him. And David Miller did yeomanry on your case. But thanks for the compliments. You're an outstanding student. You can do whatever you want. Of course, I think infectious diseases is a *great* field because there's so much you can do with it, public health, international and third world medicine, basic or

clinical research, and patient care, or combinations of all those things."
I saw a little soapbox in a corner of the examining room and climbed
on it.

"Plus, you have to maintain skills in internal medicine because many
of the patients you're asked to see don't end up having an infection. You
won't make much money, and the 'business types' will be on your case to
generate more revenue." I got off the soap box.

"By the way, I wasn't expecting you for another two to three weeks after
we'd repeated your scan. Why are you here so soon?"

"Oh, it's my parents. They wanted to see you."

"They're here in clinic?"

"Yes, waiting outside. Can we bring them in?"

"Of course. Get dressed. I'll get them from the waiting area."

Mr. and Mrs. Webb came into the examining room, holding hands
again. Alfred Webb was carrying a canvas tote bag. "Dr. Jordan, we so
much appreciated your care of Paul that we've brought you a little gift."

Four bottles of wine, two red and two white, were in the bag, all from
notable vineyards in Bordeaux and Burgundy. I'd never tasted a drop of
any of them. "Oh! You shouldn't have, these are very expensive wines."

"Not for us," he said. "I'm a wine importer. We've brought you some
nice bottles."

"Yes, I'm sure you put a lot of thought into it. I hope I can appreciate
them."

"Just enjoy them as gift of gratitude from all of us."

"You've got a special son here, you know. After today's revelations, I'm
keeping him under my wing."

———

I saw two more patients I'd recently cared for in the hospital. One was
a 22 year-old woman who had a heart valve infection related to intravenous heroin use. Her aortic valve was leaking, and she'd soon need
a valve replacement. But the cardiac surgeons were loath to operate
because the drug use invariably started up again after the surgery. The
artificial valve would then become infected, creating a situation far more

difficult to treat because of the foreign material and yet another replacement would be required. Moral dilemmas and angst ensued as to the ethical management of a patient who could not or would not cease injection drug use. And, of course, the patients never had health insurance.

The next patient had had pneumonia complicated by an accumulation of pus in the right side of her chest ("thoracic empyema"). She'd had a stormy course with hectic fevers and needed several chest tubes for drainage. She was stable now, still on an intravenous antibiotic at home.

I was nearly an hour behind. The last patient was a self-referred veterinarian with an office in Santa Monica around the corner from a British pub called *Ye Olde Queen's Head.* As I read the nurse's note in the chart, my spirits collapsed. "No! Not this morning, damn it."

"The patient states that his body is heavily infested with worms and parasites. They're coming out of his nose, his eyes and ears, his anus, and his penis." C. Peterson, R.N.

I knew right off that he had "delusions of parasitism." Patients like him often had a medical or health care background; they obsessed about worms writhing and protruding out of various orifices. They clung to their delusions, weaving complex fantasies around them. Incredible amounts of time could be spent trying to reassure the patient, usually with only transient benefit.

Psychiatrists never wanted to deal with them which I'd always found odd. I presumed that profound and cogent truths could be uncovered if someone who understood the human psyche had the inclination and determination to get to the bottom of it. Maybe that was the problem; none of my psychiatric colleagues knew much about the human psyche. They were too busy pigeon-holing patients into groups of "disorders" and syndromes, and then having arcane arguments over the bullshit they'd created.

"You look stressed out, Doctor."

I wasn't aware that I did, but maybe he had it right. Was it the body language or the look on my face? Dr. Mack Hedges, in his third and final year of training in gastroenterology, punctured my musing on the mysteries of the human psyche just as I was starting to enjoy it. Because of a shortage of faculty members in gastroenterology, Mack had been promoted early to perform scoping procedures, above and below, on patients in clinic. It was a job that needed doing, and it brought in a lot of money.

The procedure-based specialties at the University had trouble holding on to faculty members because they could make so much more money in private practice, often competing against the institution that had trained them. Hedges would leave the University in a few months to do just that. Unlike other physicians in the clinic who wore long white coats, Hedges chose an expensive suit complete with cufflinks and a silk handkerchief in his left breast pocket. To afford his attire, I presumed he was moonlighting for the gastroenterologists he'd later join in Beverly Hills.

He was a walking advertisement; it was his audition. In other words, he was "practicing to practice" in the most affluent part of the city, maybe *any* city. I had to admit though, he cut an impressive figure in clinic. He'd probably go far, admired by his wealthy patients and revered by physicians who measured success by the same yardstick.

"What? Are you obsessing again, Jordan, over a patient who's had a fever for the last six months or something?" he continued. "In all that time you spend with her, I can do any number of colon exams and be on the golf course by noon. Your problem is that you don't have an 'end organ' to probe, and probe repeatedly, I might add."

"I've never found any organ so fascinating that I wanted to think about it the rest of my life, Mack. And, I have no interest in golf."

"It's your call. Just don't complain to me that you don't make enough money."

I was eager to end the conversation, even if it meant tackling delusions of parasitism. As I resigned myself to that subject, I remembered that every patient has a story to tell. Now, I was ready for the next rendition.

"Did I ever give you my definition of the colon scope, Mack?"

"No, but you're about to, aren't you?"

"Yes. It's a long hollow tube with an asshole at both ends."

————

I knocked on the door to the examining room housing Gregory Anderson, DVM. "Good morning, Doctor. I'm Colin Jordan."

He was disheveled, unshaven, beaten up and bleary-eyed in the way of a good man gone awry I'd seen somewhere before. He was headed for skid road if we didn't break his fall. My mother's face flashed in front of me. He had a frosting of dried blood on his pants and the lower part of his shirt. On the examining table, pieces of skin floated in a specimen jar full of fluid. A dozen or so glass microscope slides were stacked up meticulously next to it.

"I'm so glad you're here to help me out, Doc," he said in plaintive monotone. "I got so damned tired of worms coming out of my penis the other night, I had to circumcise myself. I should've been circumcised when I was a boy but I wasn't for some reason. I still don't think I got them all. You will, of course, want to review the slides to verify their presence and to determine what species they are."

Scientifically trained, he had his hypothesis. Now, it only needed confirmation. "Let me check you over, Doctor. Can you get up on the examining table?"

His examination was normal except for a temperature of 102 degrees and an amateurish partial circumcision. A thick yellow-green discharge oozed from the wound margins, the onset of infection and the cause of the fever. I took the slides to the laboratory and reviewed them under a scope. I didn't expect to see anything, and I didn't, no adult worms, larvae, or eggs in the tissue, just fragments of debris.

On the way back to the room, I said to the nurse: "Carol, you should've told me right away he was this sick."

"I just went in there again, Doctor. He didn't have that specimen jar or those slides out when I put him in the room. I felt for him, I guess. I'm sorry."

"OK. Please put in a page for the urology service. Ask if they can send someone down to see him right away. He'll probably need admission for surgery."

Dr. Anderson had denied any past medical history when I first spoke to him. On further questioning, he mentioned stopping his medication a few weeks ago. "What medication was that?"

"Stelazine."

"That's a medicine for psychiatric problems. Why were you taking it, and who prescribed it for you?"

"Oh, I saw Dr. Helen Watterman, a psychiatrist in Santa Monica near my veterinary clinic for a few months, and she prescribed it. It didn't help. She didn't believe me anyway about the worms in my ears and nose. Funny thing, though. I haven't been able to sleep since I stopped taking it."

The worms had come out first in his eyes, ears, and nose, but now that he knew he needed to share his torment, they'd migrated to more intimate locations. He'd capitulated as perhaps we all do one day. I put in a call for Dr. Watterman but she was "in session". The urology service had come to see Dr. Anderson. Outside the room, the senior urologist said, "I've never seen anything quite like this. I'd like to admit him to our service for intravenous antibiotics, whatever drugs you suggest, of course. Once the infection clears up, he'll need surgery to deal with it definitively."

"I'm glad to hear you say that," but, because the infection was fairly trivial, I was more concerned about his long term psychiatric care, at least until I'd spoken to Dr.Watterman. I said:

"We should get the psych service here involved from the outset. They may want to keep him on their ward for a while after surgery. As soon as I have more information from his psychiatrist, I'll pass it on to our psychos."

I went back to the room to explain the situation to Dr. Anderson, who wanted to know, "Did you see any of them critters on the slides? " He didn't wait for an answer.

"Maybe you're doing the right thing. I guess I could use a rest."

On the way back to my office, the pager went off. "Doctor Helen Watterman here. You called?" I gave her the details.

"Yeah, I never did know what was wrong with him. The stelazine seemed to help though. Whatever you do, don't encourage anymore of this kind of behavior."

"Yeah, but what do you think about the delusions of parasitism and the……"

She'd hung up, going to her next session, I presumed. I was stunned. Didn't she care that *her* patient almost certainly in a psychotic state had mutilated himself? Was this the best she could bring herself to say? What the hell did she do with patients in her "sessions"? Put them all on stelazine, for Christ's sake! Was she on the "speaker's bureau" for the company that made the drug? Or maybe it was just the numbing effect of what psychiatrists had to deal with everyday. As I walked into the infectious diseases office, the secretary said. "You look way out of sorts. Clinic from hell?"

"Some of these frigging psychiatrists are worthless, Sue." I closed the door and sat down to dictate.

————

The Friday clinic that week was more of the same, but Emma Lazarus would have been proud of me. The first patient, a 24 year-old man, came in with a history of evening fevers to102-3 degrees, swollen lymph nodes, diffuse itching and weight loss for six months. After a look at the records, I thought he had a lymphoma, probably Hodgkin's Disease. I didn't think he had an infection but I ordered tests to rule out the likely ones such as cat scratch disease, toxoplasmosis, or brucellosis. If they were negative, I'd send him to the surgery clinic for a lymph node biopsy.

Another patient had recurrent urinary tract infections in a pattern suggesting that she had blocked drainage from one of her kidneys, maybe a stone or a tumor. The history and the organisms she had in her urine weren't consistent with a bladder infection or simple cystitis.

"Hey, Jordan!" called Mack Hedges, the budding gastroenterologist in a new and even more impressive suit. "I was thinking about your definition of the colon scope. Did you happen to see the article in this week's *New England Journal* showing the benefit of annual colon exams in men over 50 to detect early cancer? In 15 years, you'll be begging me for your exam, ready to write me a check"

"The article doesn't change a thing, Mack. Besides, another study will soon show no benefit from the exams after all the expenses. Meanwhile, gastroenterologists will fatten their wallets looking for a single colon cancer. How many colons will they perforate trying to find one?"

I called to check on Dr. Anderson, the veterinarian who'd circumcised himself. The infection around the surgical site had healed, and he was on the psychiatric inpatient service. I would go up to see him this afternoon, a social call really. His private psychiatrist, Dr. Watterman, had never phoned to check on him. Nor did she return calls from the

155

psychiatric staff at the University. She hadn't sent any medical records. "The stelazine speaker's bureau has her busy," I thought.

Paul Webb was in the imaging suite today for his follow-up CAT scan. The radiologist called me to say the study was normal except for minimal swelling on the left side of his brain, not surprising after what he'd been through. I'd see Paul one last time as a patient next week. I'd see him many times in the future as his mentor and friend though I didn't expect any more bottles of fine wine.

As I was reviewing the records on a new patient, the resident I'd worked with last month on the infectious diseases consultation service came by to see me. "Dr. Jordan, I was wondering if you'd be willing to write a letter of recommendation for my fellowship applications. I can make an appointment to see you in your office if you'd prefer. I see you're busy."

Lars Swenson was a tall handsome lad of Scandinavian stock. He had been a solid though not exceptional resident in the month we'd spent together. He had an odd ethereal quality to him. Just when you were ready to write him off as a light weight, he'd come up with a profound insight about a patient. I was already formulating in my mind what I could say in his letter. "Lars, I'd be pleased to write you a letter. Which subspecialty do you want to go into?"

"To be honest, I just want to stay here at the University. So, I'm applying in cardiology, pulmonary medicine, and renal (kidney diseases)." He was honest alright, but either incredibly naïve or deviously manipulative. He wanted a career in one of the three most lucrative fields in internal medicine. Any of them would be fine with him.

"Lars, I'm sorry. I just changed my mind. I can't write such a letter."

"You can't?"

"Think about it. The Division chiefs have a weekly meeting. They'll all know what you're up to. What am I supposed to say in this letter? Do I say that you've had a lifelong commitment to heart disease? Or do I say that you've always hankered to rescue patients suffocating from lung disease? Or is it really kidney disease that makes you go all aflutter?"

He settled on kidney disease, and I wrote a tepid letter. He got the fellowship. He probably chose nephrology because the handwriting was on the wall. Widespread use of dialysis was coming, and kidney transplants were on the horizon. Just think of all those patients with health insurance. A few years later he was still mediocre, but incredibly wealthy.

———

I knew the next patient would be a problem. With all his symptoms, he'd been referred by a family physician in Riverside, California.

When a physician, especially an internist, takes a history from a new patient, he or she goes through a defined sequence: 1) Chief Complaint – a synopsis, usually in the patient's own words, of what the symptoms are. 2) History of Present Illness - a more detailed description of the complaint, date of onset, its course, when during the day or night it occurs, how much it's bothering the patient, and so forth. 3) Past Medical History – a thorough review of previous illnesses, hospitalizations, medications, surgeries, going back to childhood. 4) Family History – details about which family members had illnesses that could be relevant to the problem at hand.

Somewhere in the sequence is the "Review of Systems," designed as a safety net to make sure all the body's systems are discussed. Through it, the physician determines whether symptoms are present the patient doesn't consider important but which may be vital in putting the puzzle together. Thus, it includes questions such as: "Have you had any problems with your eyes, ears, nose or throat? Have you been coughing, wheezing, bringing up sputum or phlegm, coughing up blood, or having any chest pain? Any problems related to your appetite, swallowing, abdominal pain, bowel movements or painful defecation? Any fever, chills, rashes, weight loss"? And so on, in considerable detail, if done right.

James Dixon was a bricklayer who'd been ill for three months. His symptoms varied daily, including fever without documentation, weight loss (estimated at thirty pounds by the patient), diarrhea with occasional bloody bowel movements, joint and muscle aches, and facial twitching, usually but not always in the left side. His physical examination by me and by all physicians before me was normal. I found no blood in his feces by chemical testing after the rectal examination.

During the review of systems, he had every symptom I asked about, a circumstance that physicians jokingly refer to as "a positive review of systems," also an indication that, almost certainly, the complaints have no physical basis. He had diarrhea and was constipated at the same time with no contradiction to him. At one point, he responded "yes" to questions about light blue bowel movements and temperatures over 108 degrees.

Exasperated, I left the room to look again at the records from Riverside. On seven office visits, his temperature had been normal, never a single fever. Mr. Dixon had gained sixteen pounds during the course of his "illness" despite his claim of weight loss. So, what was it *exactly* I was supposed to look into, a long list of complaints with no objective evidence of illness? Was it another attack by the "schizococcus? Nothing here suggested an infection or, for that matter, any medical condition.

Yet I knew that physicians in the community were under pressure to refer patients to Mecca when either the patients or their families weren't satisfied with the local ministrations. Frequently, the University consultant did provide the definitive answer in the quest to explain mysterious phenomena. But it was difficult and not often accepted by the patient, especially if it ended up being an emotional problem. A fruitless outcome could lead to appointments at yet another University or at a renowned clinic elsewhere. The quest then took on its own life with each investigation less and less likely to turn up "the" diagnosis. Nonetheless, physicians "in the trenches" of the community needed the support of their colleagues in the academic "ivory tower," the referees for all medical disagreements and mysteries.

"Mr. Dixon, I don't find much to go on here. You're medical records are benign, and your physical exam is normal. We can run more tests but I don't think anything will turn up. There's not much here to suggest you have any kind of infection. Have you been under a lot of stress lately?"

"No, nothing more than usual," he said, avoiding eye contact.

"OK, I think we should do this." I described which tests I would order and why I didn't think any would be positive. And I proposed a course of action if the tests were negative. "Most likely the problem has an emotional basis if the tests are negative, maybe from some stress you're not aware of."

Then, Mr. Dixon said, engaged now for the first time: "Doc, before you go, can I tell you something?"

"Of course, tell me anything you like. That's why you're here."

"I had sex with a bulldog."

"What's that?"

"I had sex with a bulldog about four months ago."

Now, I have to admit I was comfortable hearing just about anything from a patient. Still, this one shook me. Gathering myself, I asked. "Who did what to whom?"

"A bunch of us were sitting around a campfire drunk. One of the guys had brought along a female bulldog. They were daring me to have sex with it, so I did. Do you think that caused my medical problems?"

"In a sense, it could have, especially if you've been feeling guilty about it, but you probably didn't acquire an infection that way."

"Oh, good God! This is wonderful news, Doc! I've been feeling terrible ever since. I wish I'd said something sooner. Thank you, thank you!"

I reassured him further, shook his hand, and canceled the tests. Yet another patient had "capitulated." My next impulse was to say to Mr. Dixon, "Bless you, son. You've done right for yourself and for those who love you." I then thought, gripped in irony, "What a specialty I'd chosen, the infectious disease physician in yet another role, the shaman. Even the nut cases are fascinating. But how do I dictate the official note in a way that the patient's wife doesn't find out, his physician doesn't abandon him, and the insurance company doesn't wriggle out of some of the medical expenses? Creatively, I suppose.

I'd mention an ill-defined event that gave the patient a chance to 'turn the corner' on his way to recovery after fever, weight loss, and bloody diarrhea. No further testing would be needed. No one ever doubted a scenario like that. They were more than happy to wash their hands of it all. Maybe it was a new syndrome, and I should write it up for publication.

CHAPTER 12

CONSULTATION AND CONSOLATION

On July 1, I took over the infectious diseases consultation service, an inpatient job quite different from the one I had in May when I was in charge of a ward. Then, a group of patients lived on a floor under my control. Some of them, like Mrs. Cisneros, happened to have an infection, but most had illnesses in other areas of internal medicine. In that setting, the attending ward physician decided on the best course of action and then called the patient's private doctor outside the University with long-term recommendations. On most occasions, it was a happy time, an indication that the patient had survived Mecca.

Starting today, I would see patients all over the hospital in need of an infectious diseases consultation. The patient could be on the surgical service or on one of the surgical subspecialties like orthopedics, cardiothoracic surgery, neurosurgery, or urology; or on the neurology or psychiatric service, or even on an internal medicine ward.

I had mixed feelings about the two jobs. When serving on the internal medicine ward, I had control of what was ultimately done with the patient. The teaching opportunities for residents, interns, and medical students were broad-ranging. On the consultation service, I made recommendations on a focused aspect of patient care, but I didn't have control of what was actually done. Political and diplomatic skill was as important as medical expertise. Often, I needed to beg or cajole the medical or surgical staff to stick to a course of action. The surgeons were so busy in the operating rooms that our team had to take on broader responsibilities to make sure the patient's overall medical problems, unrelated to infection, didn't go unattended. We spent as much time dealing with fluid and electrolyte problems or abnormal liver function as we did with infection, playing center field like an anonymous gold-glove major leaguer.

The lack of control frustrated the residents rotating for a month on infectious diseases. They'd spent most of their training in charge of a group of patients, making decisions, under the supervision of an attending physician on a specific ward. On their first consultation service as we wandered all over the hospital, it wasn't uncommon for them to ask. "If they don't want to follow our recommendations, why did they call for the consultation in the first place? I don't get it!"

I usually said something like this. "Remember. We're consultants. It's their patient we're asked to see. They aren't bound to follow our suggestions verbatim though we'd like them to. Let's just be sure things make sense for the most part, and no harm is done. If the situation deteriorates, I'll call their attending physician with thinly veiled innuendo about potential medical malpractice. That usually shapes them up."

———

July 1 of each year was unique in academic medical centers. The residents who had just finished their internship now became mentors to the group of interns who arrived two or three weeks graduated from medical school. Though exaggerated, an aphorism said, "Don't get sick in July if you have to go to a teaching hospital."

Today, I was in charge of two seasoned residents and a new intern. The patients they presented were complicated, raising familiar yet still torturous dilemmas. A 37 year-old man suffered a brain hemorrhage while lifting weights at a fitness center. He collapsed with paralysis of the left side of his body. After the patient was admitted to neurosurgery with brain swelling, the surgeons inserted a tube into one of the ventricles of his brain to reduce the pressure. However, the tube became infected with a strain of staphylococcus. I recommended an intravenous antibiotic but was concerned that the tube, a foreign body, made it nearly impossible to cure the infection. In other words, the infected tube was the problem, but it had to stay in place to control the brain swelling. Time was our ally if we could get to a point of equilibrium. Then the tube could come out, and the intravenous antibiotic could be continued another four weeks at home.

We saw several patients with leukemia on the bone marrow transplant service. They shared a problem with all transplant recipients, rejection of the donor organ. Potent anti-rejection medications that suppressed the immune system were needed to keep the transplant alive. But, in addition, their nightmare was that bone marrow was the only transplant where cells from the donor attacked the tissues of the recipient to produce a disorder known as "graft-versus-host disease (GVHD)." Rejection and GVHD worked in opposite directions, each requiring toxic treatments; the patients received massive doses of immunosuppressive medications. Consequently, an astonishing array of infections developed with bacteria, fungi, parasites and viruses, particularly CMV.

Feeling inadequate, I recommended cultures, diagnostic biopsies, CAT scans, anti-infective medications, and so forth. I was disturbed as I'd always been when physicians were "causing" most of the problems with their drugs and treatments. But, in this life and death setting, they had nowhere else to turn. I knelt symbolically in homage to the oncologists. They walked that lonely "path less chosen" day in and day out.

———

The next problem was a uterus. My take on uteri was that too many of them were being surgically removed for no good reason. No one had any patience, and some doctors should have gotten an MBA instead of an MD. I was recalling a conversation I'd had with a friend, a gynecologist, after dinner in a restaurant when I asked him. "So, why do you think so many women have hysterectomies?"

"Well, they usually have back or abdominal pain. But, you know what the most common reason is? They want it taken out. They no longer have use for it after they've had children."

"Yeah, but maybe that's because the gynecologist has lead them to believe that a hysterectomy will relieve their symptoms."

"We'd never imply that," he said.

On rounds today, the new intern told me the story. The owner of the uterus in question was Katherine Blair. She'd had a cervical intra-uterine device (IUD) put in a few years ago for birth control. The device was now infected with an organism called *Actinomyces israeli,* and she had pelvic pain and a foul-smelling vaginal discharge. A normal part of the vaginal bacterial flora had sneaked in, attached to a foreign body, getting into deeper tissue. It was a rare occurrence, but every infectious diseases sleuth knew this scenario. After the intern had told me about Katherine, and we'd gone over her in detail, I said. "OK, Jennifer. When you write your note, be sure to say that Katherine needs the IUD removed followed by six weeks of intravenous penicillin. I'll arrange the home infusions and follow her in clinic. Make it clear she doesn't need a hysterectomy. Use block capital letters for that part of your recommendation. I'll say so too in my dictated note, but it'll take a day or so to get to the chart. Good that her gynecologist is a woman. The patient stands a chance."

The next day on rounds, Jennifer said. "You're won't be happy, Doctor J. Katherine Blair was taken to surgery this morning for a total hysterectomy."

What the hell was this? Female gynecologists had become misogynists just like some of their male mentors? I was shocked. I paged Dr. Ann McMahon, the surgeon. "Annie, we made it clear that Katherine Blair didn't need a hysterectomy, at least not for the infection. What was your thinking?"

"Well, she's having abdominal and back pain. Katherine's thirty-eight years old and would probably need a hysterectomy down the road anyhow; women of her age usually do. We thought we might as well do it while she was here."

Her use of the word "need" was what got to me. Katherine's only crime was that she was in the hospital. "Yeah, but the abdominal pain work-up could have waited. What was the hurry? The pain might have gone away after the infection cleared up, maybe nothing to do with her uterus. By the way, she still needs the six weeks of outpatient penicillin to take care of any remaining organisms. I'm sorry, Annie, but that was bull shit on your part."

"Don't you dare imply to her in clinic that she didn't need the hysterectomy."

"Annie, I'd never imply any such thing."

The last patient of the day might have been part of a hilarious story had not the outcome been so nearly tragic. A 49 year-old man went to buy a gift for his daughter in the charming village next to the University Hospital. She'd given birth to her first child, a girl, and his first grandchild. Strolling in the village, he twisted his ankle stepping off a curb and fell in the street. For some reason, an ambulance was called, and the attendants insisted on taking him to the Emergency Room on campus for x-rays of his ankle that was surely fractured. No, he couldn't walk there on crutches or go by wheelchair through the promenade as he wanted. He had a broken ankle.

After careening around a corner with siren blaring, the ambulance overturned and skidded a hundred feet on its roof before hitting a cemented light pole. A second ambulance was sent for and, now with three occupants, it arrived unscathed at the door of the Emergency Room. The patient and both attendants from the first ambulance were admitted to the neurosurgery service with skull fractures and other serious injuries. X-rays of the patient's ankle didn't show a fracture.

We were called because the first ambulance driver had drainage from one of his wounds that contained an organism resistant to all antibiotics tested. When I arrived on the ward, the room had been sealed around the door with iridescent chartreuse-colored tape. When I asked the nurse why, she said. "Dr. Gregorius from neurosurgery told us "not to let *that* bug out of *that* room."

After removing the tape, the infectious diseases team entered. I hadn't known that all three patients were in the same room. The beds were arranged in a "U" shape with one parallel to the window, the others perpendicular to it. Each bed held a man with limbs suspended by metal trapezes. All three patients had extensive bandages about the skull and face; it looked like a scene from a war movie or an animated cartoon.

I examined the wound in question, and it didn't look infected. A miniscule amount of fluid was draining but no pus. When a clean wound had a positive culture, it was said to be "colonized" but not infected, a common occurrence in hospitalized patients. A wound infection was defined by drainage of gross pus or inflammation at the edges. The culture then identified the cause. I wondered why anyone had bothered to culture this wound; maybe it was the July 1 effect.

I transferred the ambulance driver to a private room under wound precautions to prevent spread of the organism. Staff members and visitors now roamed in or out of his previous room as they wanted or needed to.

When I parked the car in the front of my apartment that night, I had two pages in rapid succession. Both callers were physicians wanting antibiotics that were on restricted status and required approval by the infectious diseases service. The rules had recently been put in to prevent abuse of certain antibiotics crucial in dealing with resistant bacteria and to control soaring costs. The first request was reasonable, and I approved the drug.

The second was problematic, in part because it came from a tenured associate professor who was a few years ahead of me in training at the University of Washington. He specialized in lung diseases and worked mainly in the intensive care unit. The drug he wanted to use had been studied by my colleagues and me before it was approved by the Food and Drug Administration. We'd recently added it to the hospital formulary on restricted status, requiring approval. Dr. Larry Goldman wanted to use it, but he had options, including antibiotics that weren't restricted. Knowing Larry, a "matter of principle" was at stake, and a crisis was at hand. "What the hell *is* this? I wrote an order for the drug, and the pharmacy said I had to call Colin Jordan for approval."

"It's a new program, Larry. We sent out information about it last month in the University Hospital Bulletin and in a letter to all department heads."

"What's next, for Christ's sake? I'll have to call Colin Jordan to use penicillin?"

"It just happens to be me this month because I'm on service, Larry. Next month, it's Bill Hewitt."

"This is fucking ridiculous. This isn't the University of Washington, you know, where infectious diseases run the show. Petersdorf has never worked here. It won't fly. I think any tenured faculty member should be able to prescribe whatever the hell antibiotics he wants!"

Maybe I was wrong, but I took the comment, coming from a member of the tenured faculty, which I was not, to mean that he outranked me. He'd survived the scrutiny I'd yet to see. Otherwise, what was the point of saying "tenured faculty member?"

"Does that mean you don't think instructors or assistant professors, the non-tenured faculty, can prescribe these drugs under any circumstances?"

"OK. Be a prick. I'll take this bullshit to the Hospital Executive Committee! You haven't heard the end of it, believe me."

Larry Goldman hadn't changed a bit in Los Angeles, tenure or no tenure.

———

After going to bed, I had two pages about patients on my service. I slept for an hour or so and woke up afraid that I'd given the wrong advice over the phone. When I was a resident, it wasn't unusual that, after being called during the night, I didn't remember the next day what I'd said. But as far as I knew, I hadn't made any mistakes. Now beyond that naïve certainty, I was less secure in my responses. I didn't think I'd been arrogant as a medical resident, and I was plenty humble now.

"Hi. It's Colin Jordan from infectious diseases. Did you call me an hour or so ago about Mr. Gonzalez with meningitis."

"Yes. And you recommended changing the antibiotic to vancomycin. I have the dosage you suggested here in my note."

"What was the organism again?"

"Group B streptococcus."

"And the patient had developed hives on penicillin?"

"Right. That's why I called you."

"OK. Sounds reasonable. Can you put a note in his chart to have the neurology team call infectious diseases in the morning? Thanks, and sorry to bother you."

———

When I got to the office in the morning, I had a telegram. The envelope had been opened.

Dr. Jordan:

Pleased to report your paper "Activation of Dormant Cytomegalovirus (CMV) in Mice by Immune Suppression" accepted for lectern presentation August 29, 1977.

The Selection Committee

International Herpes Virus Workshop

I'd given a number of papers at medical and scientific meetings in my young career. This one was different - not a clinical or epidemiological report but the first about my basic laboratory research, a different arena. I was to give the paper at Harvard Medical School in front of basic scientists from all over the world who worked on herpes viruses. Few physicians would be in the audience or presenting papers.

I was elated and couldn't wait to tell Bill Hewitt but, more importantly, Dr. Steven Jackson, my scientific mentor. But a great deal of work would be needed now to get the presentation in shape.

———

Before starting rounds, I went to the transcription office where my dictations for the patients seen yesterday had been typed for me to sign. Marilyn, the director of the service, said after I'd signed the notes. "I think you should have a fatherly chat with that resident of yours, Dr. Jordan."

"A fatherly chat? With which resident?"

"Dr. Glassman."

The resident in question, Dr. Frieda Glassman, had graduated first in her class at the Mt. Sinai School of Medicine in New York City. She'd just started her rotation on infectious diseases under my supervision. I thought her truly gifted and understood why she was voted "Best Intern" last year by her peers at the University. She was a dead ringer for Barbra Streisand and talked like her too. "About what, Marilyn?"

"Those white skirts she wears with no slip. Not only that, those skimpy zebra-striped or leopard-skinned panties underneath. I realize the women residents have to wear white skirts as part of their uniform, but I find the whole scene provocative and in bad taste."

"For God's sake, Marilyn! I haven't seen them because she wears a long white coat on rounds. She's an ardent feminist and president of the Association of Women House Officers. I'm only a few years older than she is. Are you nuts? I'd be crucified by the Women's Faculty Caucus. Sorry. No fatherly chat from me about this."

CHAPTER 13

FIERCE TALES AND FALSE PREMISES

Consultation rounds went in a tightly defined sequence unless we were interrupted. They had to be like that or we'd be here all night. During "sit down rounds," starting at one in the afternoon, a group of us sat at a table. An infectious diseases fellow, two residents, an intern, two or three medical students, and the attending physician made up the team.

Most of the time, at least one of the students was from another medical school, doing an elective rotation at the University Hospital. He or she was sizing up the training program, maybe hoping to land a spot for internship and residency. The competition was so fierce that the odds were against them even if they did well on this clerkship and ranked high in their class. During sit down rounds, the house staff and students presented patients for whom a consultation had been requested that day. Then, we reviewed patients seen previously. The diagnostic approach or the treatment program we'd suggested initially might need revision.

Next was a field trip to radiology to look at films and scans. Then, off to microbiology to review cultures and stains of bodily fluids. Finally, we'd wander all over the hospital to visit and examine patients. Typically, it took five or six hours. Today would take longer because we were interrupted. The resident on call took a page from the emergency room. After hearing about the patient, I didn't like the sound of it. "Warren, go down and see her. Get the lay of the land. We probably have an hour of sit down rounds still to do. Come back and present the patient to the team when you're ready."

He was back in under an hour and looked at me with tears in his eyes. "You're not going to like this, Dr. J. Are you holding on to your chair?

169

Maybe I should give you some Valium before I start. It was tough to do. I had to get the history from the patient's father who sobbed all the way through. Turns out, his wife died of cancer last year, and now he has this to deal with. My heart went out to the man. I hurried up here, but can I come back in five minutes? Sorry, I can't present her case just now."

A twenty-two year old secretary, Karen Johannsen, came to the emergency room with a dominant hemisphere stroke, meaning that the speech center on one side the brain was injured, and she was unable to speak. She had fever of 103 degrees. Two months earlier, and three weeks after a tooth extraction, she'd had fever and soreness in her finger tips while typing. Her family physician prescribed erythromycin tablets over the phone; the fever abated and her finger tip soreness disappeared. The symptoms came back a month later. This time her physician's partner prescribed tetracycline over the phone; the symptoms disappeared again. Two days before coming to the ER, the fever returned, and Karen suffered the stroke the morning she was brought in.

She had a history of rheumatic fever as a child, a disease caused by the beta hemolytic streptococcus (*Streptococcus pyogenes),* also the cause of strep throat. Rheumatic fever is complex and poorly understood, but the lasting effects involve heart valves, particularly the aortic and mitral valves on the left side of the heart. They may end up too loose and leak (aortic or mitral insufficiency) or too tight as a result of scarring (aortic or mitral stenosis). Karen had mitral stenosis where the obstructed valve blocks the flow of blood coming back from the lungs into the left ventricle. Eventually, the left atrium dilates from the strain, and blood begins to back up in the lungs. The congestion may become so severe that blood backs up all the way to the liver which then pulsates (i.e., the physician can feel the patient's pulse when palpating a tender congested liver).

Now, she was set up for another problem, infection of scarred valves, infective or bacterial endocarditis. The most common causes are two other species of streptococcus, most often, *Streptococcus viridans,* a bug we all have in our mouths. The organism enters the bloodstream and seeds the deformed heart valve often after a dental procedure. Another related bug, the enteric streptococcus (the group D enterococcus) in the gut does the same after a urinary tract infection or a procedure such as a colonoscopy.

In all forms of endocarditis, the main complications are embolic strokes caused by fragmentation of the bacterial growths ("vegetations") on the valve and further deterioration of valve function. The diagnosis can be suspected by finding so-called splinter hemorrhages under the finger and toe nails, which Karen had, rather obvious because she didn't wear nail polish. Her blood cultures, drawn in the ER, were positive for *Streptococcus viridans*.

The diagnosis of infective endocarditis is made by growing the organism from the bloodstream of a patient at risk. The physicians caring for Karen should have done the test before giving her antibiotics. Even a few doses of an oral antibiotic like erythromycin or tetracycline make it impossible to grow the organism from the blood for several weeks, but they cannot cure the infection. Treatment of endocarditis caused by *Streptococcus viridans* is either four weeks of intravenous penicillin G at a high dose or two weeks of penicillin combined with intramuscular streptomycin or gentamicin. Blood cultures should be repeated a couple of weeks after therapy to make sure there's no relapse.

Now, Karen would never move the right side of her body the same way again, and she had a facial droop. Maybe she'd recover partial speech, but she'd never speak normally. The severity of her impairment wouldn't be clear until after months of rehabilitation; it was a tragedy that could have been avoided.

After examining Karen, I left her bedside heavy of heart, thinking about her drooling and her emotion when she tried so valiantly to speak to me. Warren asked. "Is this malpractice?"

"That's a legal question, but it sure as hell was bad medicine, and I'm pissed about it. You never give a feverish patient with a history of rheumatic heart disease and an abnormal valve an antibiotic without getting blood cultures."

From his emotion in presenting Karen's case, I knew he knew, and I wanted to be sure the rest of the team would never forget. "Warren, I'd like to think that doctors in suburban LA would know better. Give me their phone number. I'll call in the morning."

I knew nothing about private practice. How would I cope with fifty patients a day clamoring at me with a litany of complaints, real and imagined? What does that do to you, and how much does it wear you down?

Yes, I took on the rawest of the raw and the most complicated patients, but what the hell did I know about private practice?

I'd never learned how to handle problems like this. No one mentioned them in medical school or residency. What's the right way to inform a physician that he or she had screwed up? At times, I was Dr. Milquetoast and sugar-coated the reprimand. At others, I flew off the handle. Today, thinking of Karen and her father, the latter was likely.

"This is Dr. Jordan in infectious diseases at the University Hospital. May I speak to Dr. Kemp about Karen Johannsen?"

I explained to him what had happened. "Yeah, I vaguely remember that day being a hassle in clinic. We must have forgotten about her mitral stenosis. Sounds like we kinda screwed up."

Before I called, I did my deep breathing exercises, afraid I might go off like a loose cannon. When the moment came, the cannon went off anyway. They'd ruined a young woman's life. "Kinda screwed up? What the hell are you talking about? You fucked up big time! She's devastated, and so is her father. Are you and your partner family physicians or internists?"

"We're both internists."

"Don't call yourself internists if this is the best you can do. You'll give the rest of us a bad name."

———

Sometimes, you can't decide what's worse; error of omission or error of commission. The last patient I saw that day was a member of a unique club I called "We tried to kill you, but you made it in spite of us." Though the club had a handful of members, their numbers were growing.

Joseph Offerman, a sixty-seven year-old Jewish accountant who played cello in a chamber music group in Ventura, had long dreamed of a trip to Israel. His favorite piece of music was "The Archduke Trio" by Beethoven, a favorite of mine as well. We had no idea when we met how the twentieth and eighteenth centuries were about to collide.

Now retired, he was thrilled to live out his dream. He had chronic lymphocytic leukemia, a relatively non-aggressive disease that comes on late in life. Still, it suppresses the immune system, making patients prone to

172

infection with certain organisms such as the pneumococcus and prone to complications if they're given a live viral vaccine.

That's what happened to Mr. Offerman. Someone in his physician's office thought he needed a smallpox booster before he left for Israel. Five days later, severe pain at the injection site came on, and he had a fever of 105 degrees with violent chills. Two days after that, an ulcer deepened at the injection site just below his left shoulder. The edges blackened, and more distant lesions typical of smallpox cropped up on his face, arms, and legs.

The diagnoses were vaccinia necrosum and disseminated vaccinia, complications of the vaccine. The more distant skin lesions told us that the vaccine virus had entered his bloodstream. Eventually, his upper left arm reddened and swelled to twice its normal size. A chest film showed bilateral patchy pneumonia. I cringed at the sight of it.

Until AIDS came along, smallpox was the greatest infectious disease scourge in the history of mankind. The virus rampaged through cities, towns, and villages, leaving a third of the populace dead and survivors deformed or scarred, especially about the face. Many were blind as well. In the 18th century, 400,000 Britons died from smallpox every year. As recently as the early 1950s, an estimated fifty million cases occurred around the world. Transmission was by inhalation of airborne droplets in the secretions of others or by inhalation of the virus inside scabbed lesions that fell off the skin of victims. Initially, pox lesions appeared on the tongue, palate or throat before the virus entered the blood stream and spread to the skin and internal organs.

Enter Dr. Edward Jenner, later Sir Edward Jenner. He was a private physician in Berkeley, a small town in Gloucestershire in the southwest of England. He'd noticed that, whenever smallpox stormed through villages, the milk maids didn't get sick. They'd already been infected by the related cowpox virus which caused pustular lesions on the nipples and udders of milking cows. The milkmaids had a mild illness that caused lesions on the hands and arms, often with low-grade fever and "minor discomfort for a brief time."

Jenner quickly tested his hypothesis. In 1796, he withdrew material from the cowpox pustules of a young milkmaid called Sarah Nelmes and injected it into the skin of an eight-year boy, James Phipps. He was the son of a worker on Jenner's grounds. He described young Phipps' reaction. "On the seventh day, he complained of uneasiness in the axilla (armpit), and on the ninth he became a bit chilly, lost his appetite, and had a slight headache. But on the tenth day he was perfectly well."

A few weeks later, Jenner challenged him by inoculating material from a smallpox victim into his skin. The injection didn't bother Phipps. Several months later, nearly two centuries before committees regulated experimentation on human subjects, Jenner challenged him again, and he didn't become ill. After a number of similar experiments, Jenner published his findings which were, of course, met with intense skepticism and derision.

But, in the end, he was right. Now, hundreds of years later, we use the terms "vaccine" and "vaccination." Both come from the Latin word for cow, *vacca*. Maybe feeling a bit guilty over "poor Phipps," Jenner had a cottage built for him and his father on the grounds.

Even Thomas Jefferson, President of the United States, was impressed, judging from a letter he sent Jenner. "Sir: I have received a copy of the evidence at large respecting the discovery of the vaccine inoculation which you have been pleased to send me, and for which I return my thanks. Having been among the early converts, in this part of the globe, to its efficiency, I took an early part in recommending it to my countrymen. I avail myself of this occasion of rendering you a portion of the tribute of gratitude due to you from the whole human family. Medicine has never before produced any single improvement of such utility. Harvey's discovery of the circulation of the blood was a beautiful addition to our knowledge of the animal economy, but on a review of the practice of medicine before or since that epoch, I do not see any great amelioration which has been derived from that discovery. You have erased from the calendar of human afflictions one of its greatest. Yours is the comfortable reflection that mankind can never forget that you have lived. Future nations will know by history only that the loathsome small-pox has existed and by you has been extirpated. Accept my fervent wishes for your health and happiness and assurances of the greatest respect and admiration.

Thomas Jefferson.

Monticello. May 14, 1806"

When I went back to Joe Offerman's room to examine him, Edward Jenner was on my mind. We still had the direct descendent of his smallpox vaccine in the form of the vaccinia virus. But by now, it had slowly become an anachronism. There hadn't been a case of indigenous small-pox in the United States since the late 1940s. By the mid-1970s, the vaccine was causing problems at a rate far greater than the miniscule risk of contracting smallpox, at least in the US.

Too many people with weak immune systems like Mr. Offerman's were vaccinated and suffered life-threatening complications. The notion of repeatedly vaccinating people with genital herpes to create some vague form of "viral interference" had taken hold, causing problems far worse than genital herpes. Routine immunization of Americans against small-pox was abandoned. The disease was eradicated globally in 1979, thanks to Sir Edward Jenner. His insight nearly two hundred years earlier was the greatest achievement in the history of public health.

"Joe, did you know that Beethoven and Mozart both had mild cases of smallpox?"

He wasn't interested in them this afternoon. "Doc, am I going to make it to Israel alive or not? I have a cemetery plot there in either case."

I didn't know, but we did what we could to control his leukemia and his infection, using an experimental anti-viral drug called methisazone. He was one of the first patients to receive it. I don't know if it did any good, but we nearly wiped out his liver using it. Still, six months later, he was in Jerusalem under his own power.

On his last day in the hospital, he entertained the staff and patients in the lounge with an impassioned rendition on the cello of the solo parts of Tchaikovsky's whimsical "Variations on a Rococo Theme." As I applauded, he grinned broadly to a standing ovation, grateful to be alive I thought.

When I reviewed the photocopied records from the office of Joe's physician, I couldn't tell why the smallpox vaccine had been given or whose idea it was. A page was missing. I called the office, and the physician was on vacation. The nurse I spoke to said. "It's my understanding that the Israeli government requires a smallpox vaccination within the year prior to a person entering the country."

"Yes, but countries usually wave the requirement if the physician writes a letter saying that the vaccine is contraindicated because of an underlying condition."

"Let me look into it and call you back."

A few hours later she paged me. "I'm sorry, Doctor. I was the one who photocopied the records we sent you. You have a missing page because we have a missing page. I don't know whose idea it was to offer Mr. Offerman smallpox vaccine."

The smallpox virus, the vaccine, and I ran into each other now and again. Twenty-five years after I'd taken care of Joe Offerman, I was working in Portland at the Oregon Health & Science University, just a year or so after the September 11 terrorist attacks. Letters laced with the anthrax bacillus were being sent to senators and media personalities. Bioterrorism preoccupied many of my colleagues in infectious diseases around the country. Much of it was self-serving in the hope that the federal government would fund research to address the problem or maybe my colleagues could promote themselves. At national meetings during special sessions on bioterrorism, one of the rabble rousers invariably hollered from the top of the auditorium. "We are not prepared! We'd better get a plan people!"

The voices of reason were oddly silent, perhaps afraid to be wrong. Islamic fundamentalist women, akin to suicide bombers, might infiltrate the perfume counters of Macy's department store armed with seductive aromatic sprayers full of the anthrax bacillus or the smallpox virus. I worried more about massive bombs going off in congested public places.

With this in mind, I reluctantly agreed to give an interview on smallpox as a weapon to a reporter from a local television station in Portland. Mary Keller was sincere enough on the phone, but I'd done enough media interviews to know that a land mine might be on the horizon. Still, maybe I could use the interview as a chance to educate people and quell the hysteria.

Mary introduced me to the camera man and explained what sort of questions she'd be asking. It all went out the window once the green light blinked on the camera. The pitch of her speech went up half an octave and so did the decibel level. "Smallpox, Doctor, scary isn't it? Aren't you scared?"

I shouldn't have been taken aback by the tone of the initial salvo, but I was. After a moment to collect myself, I said "No, I'm not scared, but I have some concerns."

"We all do, Doctor. What concerns you the most?"

"Well, we stopped routinely vaccinating for smallpox just over twenty-five years ago. So, younger people are not immune. If there were a terrorist incident, they'd have the highest priority for vaccination. We'd have to quickly mobilize our public health resources."

"Precisely, and that's what worries me, especially after all the recent funding cuts to the public health infrastructure by states and the federal government."

"The federal government is earmarking funds for just this purpose. We'll be up to speed soon."

"But do you trust the federal government to be in charge of anything this important?"

"Yes, I do, meaning the Centers for Disease Control and the National Institutes of Health. They're the best in the world in dealing with something like this. Who do you want in charge, corporate America?"

Her semi-hysterical tone continued with more alarmist questions and statements. After she indicated the end of the interview was near, I said. "Mary, I think it's important for the viewers to know that if we can eradicate smallpox from the globe as we did more than twenty years ago, including the control of it under the most primitive conditions in Africa and elsewhere, we can deal with it at home."

When I saw the interview on television that evening, the last sentence was left out. A diatribe by Ms. Keller about the "appallingly vulnerable state of our people in the twenty-first century" aired instead. She didn't say anything about how many "vulnerable people" like Joe Offerman would have died if we'd kept vaccinating them against a disease that no longer existed, at least not on this planet. Never let me do a television interview again.

———

Sometimes we harm patients when a naive attending physician assumes that the residents know more than they do, a mistake he allows himself once a career. Learning never stops.

During my first year as a faculty member and attending physician at the University Hospital, we admitted Matt Rollins to the internal medicine ward. He was a homeless man, probably an alcoholic, who came in with low grade fever, thirty pound weight loss over six months, and pain in the right chest whenever he took a breath or coughed. His physical examination was noteworthy for badly decayed teeth and dullness to percussion over the lower right half of his chest. His breath sounds were inaudible in the same area. The findings suggested that he had a significant amount of fluid there, and the x-ray confirmed the physical findings. He also had a positive skin test for tuberculosis.

After she'd presented the patient on rounds, the resident, Paula Shields, said to me. "We'll do the thoracentesis this afternoon to get a look at the fluid and for a culture." A thoracentesis is a tap of the chest to obtain fluid for analysis. I said, "Yes, of course, but since tuberculous pleurisy is in the running, he also needs a pleural biopsy. Have you ever done one with a Cope needle?"

"I should've thought of that. I've done several. And I'm a whiz with the Cope needle."

"Well, Mr. Rollins is in good hands then."

The Cope needle is a device with a little hook on the end that allows the physician to snag a small piece of pleura, the membrane lining the chest and the lungs. Biopsy is especially important in tuberculous pleurisy because the characteristic inflammation (granulomatous inflammation) and the typical organisms are not usually free in the fluid, and the stains and cultures are rarely positive. You find what you need for diagnosis in the pleural tissue, not in the fluid. OK, then, everything was kosher with Mr. Rollins, and we were good to go.

Later that afternoon, as I dictated his note, I thought about his carious teeth. I'd failed to mention to the house staff that an anaerobic infection due to aspiration of putrid oral secretions into his lungs, especially in an alcoholic with lapses of consciousness, was in the differential diagnosis. But surely they knew that, didn't they? To keep my dictation up to the moment, I paged Dr. Shields. "What do we know about the pleural fluid on Mr. Rollins?"

"It was gross pus, and it smelled terrible, all putrid like.

"OK, so it's an anaerobic infection due to his rotten teeth and not tuberculosis. You didn't do the Cope biopsy once you knew that, right?"

"No, we went ahead with it. Should we not have?"

"Oh, shit," I thought, ready to blame Paula, a Harvard medical graduate who'd spent time at the Boston City Hospital where she'd probably seen plenty of patients like Mr. Rollins. But no, it was me, Dr. Idiot, the attending physician, who'd been in charge, and I'd failed to remind her of what I assumed she knew. Never assume anything in medicine even if it means you'll be a pain in the ass for residents and your colleagues for years. "Paula, have Mr. Rollins lie prone for the rest of the day and as much of the night as he can. Put iced compresses every hour on the back of his right chest where the biopsy was done."

The next morning, the back of him looked like the right half of Quasimodo, the Hunchback of Notre Dame; poor Mr. Rollins. His back was puffed out due to pus seeping through the hole in the pleura made by the biopsy needle. He was taken to surgery, and his back was filleted for about a foot. I never made that mistake again. But what mistake I hadn't thought of was just around the corner?

———

Not only may physicians occasionally harm patients, they sometimes harm themselves. James Carmody was a retired obstetrician-gynecologist, seventy-four years old. At one time, he'd been chairman of the OB-GYN department. Currently, his son Patrick was the chairman. I guess leadership ran in the family.

Jim Carmody developed shingles or zoster involving a skin dermatome on the right side of his chest. Shingles, of course, is a common occurrence in the elderly, coming on in about fifteen percent of people past the age of seventy. Yet another deceitful herpes virus took its revenge after chicken pox in childhood set up the dormant infection in nerve cells.

Unfortunately, Jim knew a little something about anti-viral drugs. He called the pharmacy on the ground level of his high rise apartment building. The prescription was for the drug acyclovir which is used to treat oral and genital herpes simplex virus as well as varicella-zoster virus (VZV) infections. To treat herpes simplex, the dose was around a gram a day divided into five doses. To treat shingles, the dose was much higher because VZV was not as sensitive to the drug; it required a dose around four grams a day. But Jim had forgotten or perhaps never knew that acyclovir was excreted by the kidneys. He'd had poor kidney function for years because of hypertension and diabetes.

Five days later, he came to the ER disoriented and combative. He took a swing at a male nurse of Asian descent in the ER calling him "a filthy cheating spy." Carmody had been an intelligence officer in the US Army in the Pacific during World War II. He was promptly sedated and sent up to the ward. Now he was our problem.

When my resident and I reviewed his case, we couldn't sort out the three most likely possibilities for his confusion. He had brain toxicity, the most common side effect of too much acyclovir. He had encephalitis because of the zoster infection. Or the confusion was due to a combination of those events aggravated by sedation. First and foremost, we needed spinal fluid to make sure it wasn't encephalitis which would require high dose intravenous acyclovir.

But the spinal fluid didn't come easy. No, it didn't come at all. He'd had so many back surgeries that my resident and I couldn't get the needle into his subarachnoid space. After we'd given up, I said. "OK Allen, let's take him down to radiology and see if they can get in under fluoroscopic x-ray guidance. Or maybe they can do a cisternal tap at the base of his skull."

We'd had him on his left side for about an hour while we tried to do the lumbar puncture. When we rolled him over to move him onto a gurney, another problem cropped up. The entire left side of his body was black with necrotic skin, and his temperature was now 105 degrees. It took us a couple of days to sort it out when the blood cultures came back positive for the Group A beta-hemolytic streptococcus. As a complication of his shingles, he had what was called by the tabloids "the flesh-eating virus" even though it was not a virus, again the same bacterium that caused rheumatic fever and strep throat. The condition, necrotizing fasciitis, had been reported in medical journals for the first time a few months earlier.

What followed was frenzy. The left side of his body was filleted from head to toe, and he eventually lost his left leg, disarticulated at the hip. When we at last got a look at his spinal fluid, there was no evidence of encephalitis from VZV. The only way we could put it together was that he had acyclovir nervous system toxicity in an attempt to self-treat his shingles. That had been followed by the streptococcus entering his blood stream through one or more of his shingles skin vesicles. The reason that the left side of his body had gone dead was because of our insistence on having him lie there while we tried to get spinal fluid. Bacteria in the blood stream like to home in on traumatized or pressured parts of the body.

I couldn't sleep a few nights, dreaming of Dr. Carmody's charred and mutilated body having rigors on its bed as we stubbornly went after spinal fluid. And I had dreams that I'd not yet seen the horror that infectious diseases might bring all of us. The dreams weren't exaggerating. Yes, we had antibiotics, and yes we had vaccines. But new infections would never stop coming.

———

For two of those years at the University Hospital, we had a post-doctoral fellow who'd done his residency in internal medicine in Madrid. Accepting an applicant from a foreign country was a roll of the dice. You might've hired a gem with something to prove or you might've hired your worst nightmare. Our division chief Bill Hewitt made the right call in the case of Emilio Rodriquez, pronounced Rodrigueth in Castilian Spanish. When he returned to Spain, he was the country's first infectious disease specialist to train in the United States, and he went on to a career of distinction.

The first day we went on rounds together, I was glad to have him. Many of our consultations involved Mexican patients who didn't speak English, and my Spanish was primitive. Emilio had rather thick glasses that exaggerated the size of his pupils. When I asked him to translate what a patient had just told us, he looked at me with pupils twice their normal size. "I have never heard such Spanish in all my life," he said.

"Is it crude?"

"No, it's beautiful, but she's speaking to us from the eighteenth century."

———

As bad as it is that physicians occasionally harm patients from lack of knowledge or poor judgment, nothing infuriates me more than sleazy medicine by money-hungry doctors. Later that day, we got a page from ophthalmology about a patient with pain and loss of vision in his right eye and a temperature of 105 degrees. They suspected bacterial endophthalmitis, a sight-threatening infection involving the inner membranes of the eye, and he was going to surgery for drainage.

The patient was Nathan Green, a well-known "show business" attorney from Beverly Hills. His course had been so tumultuous that no one had

181

had a chance to take a proper history. In the operating room, just as the ophthalmologists were preparing to drain the eye, the globe (eyeball) ruptured, and pus under pressure poured forth.

Emilio and I spent much of the evening taking his history, after he woke up from anesthesia and learned that he'd lost his right eye. Before we went into the room, the ophthalmology resident had warned us. "Be careful. He's very upset as you might expect. I have no idea how the hell this happened. He's frustrated, just a word of warning."

Mr. Green had been receiving twice weekly "chelation therapy" for persistent anxiety. Numerous intravenous infusions of a solution containing EDTA (ethylene diamine tetra-acetic acid) were given to "to remove divalent cations such as calcium and iron from his system." The treatment was bogus; nothing indicated that it was effective for anxiety or any medical condition. Still, it was widely used, especially in Hollywood. That was the location of Dr. Mohammed Ahmed's practice. He was Nathan Green's doctor.

The next day, we had the results of the cultures on Mr. Green. The pus from the ocular globe, his blood, and his urine were all growing *Bacillus cereus*, a Gram-positive rod better known for causing food poisoning after the ingestion of spoiled meat. The organism wasn't recognized as a cause of bacterial endophthalmitis at the time. I presumed that his infection had resulted from bacterial contamination of the EDTA infusions.

When I called Dr. Ahmed to explain what had happened to Nathan Green, he said with a thick accent. "I am so sorry to hear this. It has nothing to do with the chelation therapy, of course. We've never had a problem with it."

"It has everything to do with your horseshit therapy if you can call it that," I was thinking. "You don't get a disseminated *Bacillus cereus* infection out of the blue." Then I said. "You may be right, but do you mind if we come to your office to pick up a few of the vials of EDTA that were used to treat Mr. Green?"

I was shocked when Ahmed agreed to let us pick up the vials. When I got to his office, I found out that the staff used multi-dose vials that required repeated needle aspirations to withdraw the EDTA used on different patients. That's probably how the bacterial contamination occurred. How many other patients had been infected? Ahmed's practice offered nothing other than chelation therapy. He hadn't taken a history or examined a patient in years.

The cultures of both vials of EDTA grew out a strain of *Bacillus cereus* identical to the one that caused Nathan Green to lose his right eye. I turned the information over to the Los Angeles County Health Department. The epidemiologist said they were overwhelmed at the moment but would look into it as soon as they could. Then, I presented my findings to Mr. Green, who was looking at me with a patch over one eye socket. He said, "it's partly my fault, damn it! I have a lot of nutty friends in entertainment. I probably shouldn't have listened to them about this crap. But I know, believe me, what to do with fucking Dr. Ahmed. He'll think it was 'an eye for an eye.' The guy's probably making mega-bucks with his expensive treatments that aren't covered by insurance. They're considered experimental, cash up front, you know. Would you be willing to testify against him as an expert witness?"

I thought about that one for a moment. "I don't think it would be a good idea."

"Why not?"

"It might come across as collusion between us since I was one of your doctors. I'm presenting your case at the infectious diseases conference this week. A number of doctors in our department will know about you. Any one of them could handle it, and they know their way around a court room better than I do."

Practicing medicine is exacting, enthralling, exhilarating, enlightening, and, inevitably, damned frustrating. The risk of a screw-up is far greater when the doctor's field is broad. Maybe we've placed too great a burden on physicians in primary care. Maybe that's why only a few intrepid souls wanted to do it when the twenty-first century dawned. It's easier for a specialist to survive performing the same procedures over and again, though he's still at risk.

I don't respect or condone lack of knowledge, poor judgment, or incompetence. And I know any physician's worst nightmare might strike on a brutal day in clinic when it all goes wrong in spite of impeccable judgment and a high degree of skill. But those foibles don't come from the same font in the soul as deceit and avarice. I wanted Dr. Ahmed and his "practice" wiped off the face of the earth.

The Health Department got around to checking into Mr. Green's case about two weeks later. They came to the same conclusion even though the remaining vials of EDTA had disappeared from his office by then. Fortunately, I had the data. Nathan Green went after Dr. Ahmed in court, and his practice was shut down.

Because of the unusual organism causing Mr. Green's infection, Emilio and I decided to write his case up for publication. It turned out over the next ten years that, for some reason, *Bacillus cereus* would become well-known as the most common cause of bacterial endophthalmitis. When Emilio gave me the first draft of the manuscript, I knew I was in for a *tour de force.* The first sentence read, "Bacterial endophthalmitis is one of the eye's most fearful penetrating traumatisms."

––––––

The aphorism from the 1980s that "herpes is forever" has some truth to it. When herpes simplex virus initially enters the body through a mucous membrane or the skin, it penetrates the terminal nerve endings providing sensation to the site. The virus then migrates through the axoplasm (the cytoplasm of the nerve trunks) until it reaches the nucleus or brain trust of the nerve cell, the neuron.

If the virus enters through the mouth, the eye, or the facial skin (usually HSV-I), it migrates to the neurons in the trigeminal ganglia which are located behind each eye. If it's introduced into the genital mucosa or skin (usually HSV-II), the virus ends up in the neurons of the paraspinal ganglia alongside the spinal column. Once inside the neurons at either site, HSV establishes a latent or non-replicating infection. It's important to understand that the latent virus does not replicate because anti-viral therapy can only inhibit replicating viruses.

Most often, the initial or "primary" infection with HSV at either site is completely asymptomatic. We know this because eighty-five percent of the population has antibodies against HSV-I (indicating prior infection), yet only fifteen percent has ever had a "cold-sore" or fever blister. Occasionally, a person with a primary HSV-I infection will develop a mouthful of ulcers ("primary herpetic stomatitis") with high fevers and swollen lymph nodes in the neck. They may need to be hospitalized because they cannot eat or take in fluids. Similarly, a patient with a primary HSV-II genital infection may develop high fevers with viral invasion of the blood stream, sometimes resulting in viral meningitis.

What happens after the initial infection varies greatly. The recurrent lesions that occur in some people result from a reverse of the viral entry process. In other words, the virus migrates out of the neuronal nucleus into the axoplasm and takes the same forks in the road it used to enter the cell initially. Once the virus reaches the mucous membrane or the skin, it produces lesions at the same sites over and over again. Infected patients can usually predict when they are about to develop lesions because the virus causes nerve malfunction as it migrates down the axon. The patient senses burning or stinging discomfort before the virus arrives at the skin or mucous membrane.

A number of well-known stimuli cause the virus to reactivate. For both HSV-I and HSV-II, emotional stress is a common trigger. For type I, the other common stimuli are sunlight and fever (hence the term "fever blister"). Sunlight probably irritates the terminal nerved endings in the skin which presumably send an "activation signal" to the virus dormant in the neuron. Some of the worst fever blisters are seen among skiers, presumably because of the dual nerve triggers of sunlight and windburn.

When a patient has his or her first set of lesions, they may be from a first or primary infection or caused by virus that has been dormant in nerve cells for years. It's important for physicians to know this when one partner in a committed relationship develops genital lesions for the first time; it doesn't necessarily indicate infidelity. We can also use this fact to get someone off the hook if we're so inclined.

The frequency with which a person develops lesions after the initial infection varies greatly over time. For about thirty consecutive years, I developed a cold-sore in the middle of my upper lip every year between Christmas and New Years. About ten years ago, they stopped visiting, maybe because I'd learned how to handle the stress as I got older.

A particularly troublesome form of HSV-I infection is herpetic whitlow, lesions occurring on one or more fingers. Invariably, it occurs in medical or dental workers who frequently suction or have contact with saliva or respiratory secretions of patients. Painful redness and swelling of the digit develops with a tender swollen lymph node in the armpit on the same side as the affected digit. A few days later, typical HSV vesicles erupt on the surface of the red swollen finger.

The trouble comes when the patient goes to the ER before vesicles appear on the finger. Many physicians aren't familiar with whitlow, and they assume the problem is due to streptococcal pyoderma or a staphylococcal infection. They incise the finger with a scalpel expecting to find pus, but there isn't any. Now, HSV enters more nerve endings that have been exposed by the procedure and recurs more frequently that it would have if nothing had been done.

Cassie Milton was a twenty-six year-old nurse on the pediatric bone marrow transplant ward. She was referred to me by a colleague in pediatric infectious diseases who said, "I don't get it. She's had six episodes of zoster (shingles) over the last year despite high dose acyclovir. She's a great nurse. It's a sad situation. I've kinda taken her under my wing. She had a child out of wedlock just over a year ago. The kid has cerebral palsy. I checked out Cassie's immune system, and it's normal. It just doesn't add up."

"Where are the lesions located?"

"They always occur in the lower back and involve the upper part of her left buttock. They're very painful."

"Sounds more like HSV-II to me."

"HSV-II occurs on the buttocks?"

"Yeah, one of its favorite sites."

Oh, these naïve pediatricians, bless them. Shingles, caused by reactivation of the varicella-zoster virus (VZV) decades after a bout of chicken pox, is not a recurrent disease in people with normal immune systems.

"Ted, let's do this. Stop the acyclovir, and let the lesions come on sooner than later. Ask her to call me the next time she has them, and I'll see her in clinic."

A month later, Cassie called me. She had lesions on the left buttock as usual. I aspirated one of the vesicles with a needle and sent the fluid for viral culture. It grew HSV-II, but there was more to it than that.

Fifteen months earlier, she'd gone into labor prematurely because she had viral meningitis with high fever and shaking chills. I wondered if it wasn't a bout of primary infection with HSV-II. Before then, she'd never had herpetic lesions on her buttock. At birth, her daughter was normal. There was no mention in the records I could get from Methodist Hospital whether Cassie had genital lesions due to HSV-II at the time of delivery. Calls for further information were ignored. Cerebral palsy it wasn't.

A week after she was born, Cassie's daughter, Chelsea, had the sudden onset of vesicles on her face and left hand. A day later, she an epileptic fit and was rushed to the hospital. The infant was treated with intravenous acyclovir after HSV-II was grown from her blood and the vesicle fluid. After the hospitalization, Chelsea "was never the same" according to Cassie.

If a pregnant woman has active genital lesions due to HSV at the time of vaginal delivery, fifty percent of the newborns will acquire the infection as they pass through the birth canal. Of those, half will die, and many of the survivors end up devastated with central nervous system complications. A Caesarean section should be done to protect the newborn.

I'd never been an advocate of medical malpractice suits with aggrieved patients and avaricious lawyers going after doctors who'd tried to do their best. Medicine is too complicated, too hard, and it's too easy to fail for all the right reasons. I'm not talking about sponges or surgical instruments being left in a patient's belly or the wrong leg being amputated, but I am talking about a cover-up.

I'd called medical records at Methodist several times to get information. The last time I called I said to the person at the other end of the phone. "OK, if you're not going to send me the records for some reason, can I make an appointment to come by and look at them?"

"Are you on the medical staff or do you have privileges here?" she asked.

"No, I don't."

"Then, no, you can't just waltz in here. By the way, I tried to respond to your initial request for the records, but they are missing."

Cassie continued to have lesions every month or so. I changed antiviral medications, but it didn't help. On one of her visits, I had a medical student working with me who asked off-handedly. "Does she go to the tanning booth? Does she have that tan all year?"

I was Dr. Idiot again. Though I'd never heard of HSV-II activated by sunlight or, in this case, artificial sunlight, no reason said it couldn't be. And Cassie's lesions occurred just above the bottom half of the bikini she wore in the tanning booth. I asked her to stop going for three months. She had no lesions afterward. In fact, she had no lesions over the three years I followed her, even after I stopped her antiviral medication.

The most torturous decision I had to make on Cassie was whether to tell her about a possible primary HSV-II infection at the end of her pregnancy. We needed to find out if she'd had genital lesions at the time of vaginal delivery, indicating the need for a Caesarian section.

Maybe she was better off believing Chelsea had cerebral palsy. Could she come to grips with another story; she'd had primary genital herpes late in pregnancy and her infection was responsible for the child's developmental delay, probable mental retardation, and seizure disorder? After a few weeks of caring for Cassie and stewing about it, I thought she should know. Otherwise, wouldn't I'd be part of the collusion and cover up? "Let's go after the sons-a-bitches if that's what they are," I thought.

She looked radiant and studious in her glasses today with a smile to warm your heart. According to my colleague in pediatrics, "She's the most loving nurse we have when it comes to kids with leukemia. We can't let bad things happen to her."

"Cassie, to be certain, we need a look at your medical records. We could hire a malpractice attorney on a contingency basis to subpoena them. I'll help you. It could be a way to pay for Chelsea's medical expenses. I think we should at least try to get to the bottom of it." Maybe with the best of intentions, I'd overplayed my hand, a vigilante let loose.

After a moment, her face flushed, and the tears came. "Oh, I don't know, Doctor, if I want to deal with this anymore. It's been dreadful. Let me think about it. Maybe we should just let the sleeping dog lie."

"OK. Call me if you want to discuss it further."

———

That was the year I was appointed chairman of the intern selection committee for the Department of Internal Medicine, a thankless task. The Department had more than a thousand applicants for twenty-eight internship positions. A computerized system called the National Intern-Resident Matching Program matched candidates and hospitals. The applicants ranked the hospitals they wanted in order of preference. The hospitals did the same with the candidates. The results were given to candidates and hospitals on a fateful day in April before internship started in July.

Jubilation and profanity erupted in medical school hallways all over the country on that day. Despite being advised against it, some applicants listed programs they really didn't want or cities where they really didn't want to live. They did so to make sure they didn't end up "unmatched" after the results came out. The pickings were slim if a student didn't match. Invariably, more than a few candidates who opened their envelopes on match day were not happy.

I was responsible for making sure that the candidates had an interview by a member of the committee, that they met at least one resident currently in the program, and that lunch for all the candidates was available on any given day. A secretary was assigned to help me, but something always went wrong, usually when I was in the middle of rounds.

The committee meetings started out amicably enough, but as time wore on they became more contentious. Each member had his or her own take on what we should do. At one meeting, a cardiologist said: "Look, I'm tired of all these geniuses, the interns who know everything about the urine calcium or the serum porcelain concentrations, but can't talk to a patient or his family without pissing them off. Let's emphasize how the candidate comes across during the interview more than where he ranks in his class. To put it simply, let's get some nice guys, for Christ's sake."

At another, an arrogant Ivy League snob, said with a sneer. "I don't know about the rest of you, but I would take the bottom student in the class at Cornell over the top student from Illinois or Michigan anytime."

We all got better reading letters of recommendation from each applicant's medical school. It helped to compare the letters for students attending the same medical school, looking at the subtleties and nuances or even red flags in the carefully chosen verbiage. It was also helpful to review the letters of last year's applicants who were now our interns. We knew how well they'd worked out or not. No matter how strong the applicant pool seemed or what we did, at least one catastrophe matched to our program every year, someone who'd never mastered the history and physical exam or someone who couldn't see the forest for the trees, running up the patient's hospital bill with too many tests.

We also figured out that a summary statement at the end of a letter from a certain Ivy League medical school meant that the student was in the bottom third of his class if it said he was a "very good candidate," instead of an "outstanding" or "excellent candidate." One private medical school in Chicago thought so highly of its students that all letters included the statement: "Please note that our University draws from the best of the best medical school applicants around the country. Take this into account when comparing them to students from lesser medical schools." Even so, we'd never had an intern who was any better than average from that school.

In February, I interviewed my last candidate for the year, a woman from Duke University School of Medicine in North Carolina. Maybe feeling a bit wistful, my thoughts drifted back to interviews I'd had when applying for internship. My first was at Stanford University. The professor interviewing me was renowned for coming up with a cure for Hodgkin's Disease, using a combination of chemotherapy and radiation. After welcoming me to Stanford, he asked me with a sardonic grin on his face. "Can you name five circumstances where a patient might have elevated vitamin B-12 levels in his blood?"

I was taken aback in the first moments of the interview, though Stanford had a reputation for this. Still, it irritated the hell out of me. "Yes, I think I can if you allow me to list each of the myeloproliferative disorders separately."

"Go on, then," the professor said.

"Well, then you would have polycythemia rubra vera, essential thrombocytosis, myelofibrosis, and chronic myelogenous leukemia. The fifth cause would be two many vitamin B-12 shots, probably for no good reason."

"You know, you're the first student who's ever answered that question."

"Well, you see, I intend to specialize in minutia."

My next stop was at U.C.L.A Medical Center in Westwood, Los Angeles. Again, I was interviewed by a hematologist. He was a supercilious ass. He said, "Personally, I don't think anyone should intern in a University Hospital. There's too much specialization. For a really varied internship experience, you should train in a general hospital as I did."

Then, he turned a hundred and eighty degrees to point out his internship certificate on the wall. It was from the Massachusetts General Hospital, the most prestigious hospital in the country, maybe the world. I guess he wanted me to know he'd been a hotshot. I responded, "yes, but I know the University Hospital here functions as the county hospital for

West Los Angeles and the San Fernando Valley. We should have a lot of general hospital patients."

"Son, good luck wherever you go. To be honest, I haven't rounded on the wards here in years. I have no idea about our patients anymore."

The third stop on the interview trail was the University of Washington Hospitals in Seattle. I fell in love with the place, and some of it had to do with the interview. I met a professor who ran the division of nuclear medicine which was new but up and coming. He said to me. "I know these interviews are hectic and stressful. Half the time, you guys don't get lunch. My wife made us a chicken sandwich, and I have a couple of cold ones in the fridge. Let's go sit on the grass by the Lake Washington ship canal. We can talk there."

———

Interviewing my last candidate that season, I gradually began to lose vision on the left side of the retina in both eyes, so called "homonymous hemianopsia." I could only see the right half of the visual field with each eye. I was convinced I had a brain tumor. George Gershwin and Frau Feldman's husband came to mind, though I hadn't yet smelled burnt rubber or natural gas.

To maintain eye contact with the candidate, I tilted my head forty-five degrees to the right. She must have thought me odd, and I imagined her thinking, "What a creep, leering at me! How the hell did this guy become chairman of the intern selection committee?"

After the interview, I wanted to report for a CAT scan, thinking I had a tumor in the left visual tract of my brain. What else could it be? Later, a dull headache started at the back of my head on the left, and I had wavy scintillations in both eyes like fumes rising from asphalt on a hot day. I took six hundred milligrams of ibuprofen, and everything was gone in an hour. It had been the aura of a classic migraine headache, and I'd blown the diagnosis in its early moments. Nowadays, I always carry four hundred milligrams of ibuprofen with me to nip it in the bud before it gets to the headache stage. Later on, when I was chief of infectious diseases at the University of Minnesota, the winter sun bouncing off ice and snow set the visual symptoms off like clock work, especially on days when the sky was clear as a bell, and it was thirty below zero.

———

The committee finished its work after much dissension and acrimony. We ranked about one hundred of the eleven hundred applicants. I took our final rank list to Dr. David Gordon's office for his signature. He was the chairman of the Department of Internal Medicine. A few days later, his secretary called me. "When you have a moment, drop by the office and sign the final rank order before we send it to the national matching program. You need to sign it as chairman of the committee. Dr. Gordon thanks you and the committee for doing an outstanding job."

When I saw the final list, I didn't recognize it. The student now ranked number one was one of our own in the bottom third of the class. We hadn't ranked him. His family had donated the land on which the University Hospital had been built. Several more of our own students followed on the list. The committee hadn't ranked any of them. The student from the University of Pennsylvania we'd listed number one was now number thirteen.

When I got back to my office, I called another member of the committee and told her what had happened. She said in a matter of fact tone. "Well, he's the chairman. I guess he can do whatever the hell he wants."

I wasn't taking it with the same equanimity, maybe because I'd done eighty percent of the committee's work. I made an appointment the next day with Dr. Gordon to complain. He said, "I don't understand why you're so upset. Didn't I say when I appointed you to chair the committee that it was strictly advisory to the chairman?"

"No you didn't, Dave. If you had, I wouldn't have done it."

I resigned as chairman, but continued to serve on the committee.

CHAPTER 14

EXCELLENCE IS EXCELLENCE

Steven Jackson, D.V.M., Ph.D., was a brilliant scientist, referring to himself now and then as a "hard-nosed S.O.B.". He'd graduated from veterinary school and later had taken a Ph.D. in microbiology at the University of Washington in Seattle. When he joined the faculty at the University in Los Angeles, the work he did on herpes viruses of swine and cattle was elegant. The experiments probed the mechanisms involved in replication of viruses in cells and the effects the viruses had on cell function. Other scientists were doing similar experiments on herpes viruses of animals, amphibians, and humans, just a step or two behind Jackson.

On top of that, he had a vicious hand-ball game, keeping his hostile impulses in check, he'd told me. He was a genius. At his epiphany, he recognized the edge he had to do research few others could. Yes, he was a sophisticated virologist and molecular biologist. But Steven had a handle on diseases as a veterinarian that other Ph.D. scientists didn't. Once he pulled it together, he made monumental contributions on the role of viral infections in human and animal diseases. Over the next few years, he opened enough avenues of research to keep other scientists going for decades.

I first learned of Jackson's research when a paper came out in the journal *Science* in 1971. I was at the Centers for Disease Control. In the paper, Jackson and his colleague, Dr. Barbara Covington, had developed in mice a model showing that herpes simplex virus hid from the immune system in the nucleus of nerve cells or neurons. Genital lesions were skyrocketing in the general population at the time. Jackson's work had gotten the attention of physicians and the public.

The virus also caused two other devastating problems: encephalitis with a 60% death rate in otherwise healthy adults (the diagnosis suspected by Dr. David Miller in the illness of our medical student, Paul Webb) and a disseminated infection in newborns with a similar death rate (the scenario in the case of Cassie Milton and her daughter Chelsea). The finding that neurons harbored the virus was what we needed to explain a mystery. How did the virus cause lesions at the same site over and again on the oral or genital mucosa, the cornea, or the skin?

Because of Jackson, I wanted a position at the University Hospital though none had been advertised. I was delighted when Bill Hewitt called me to interview and to give a research seminar. The implication was that it might be possible to pull together a position if there were sufficient funds and interest among the relevant parties. The timing of my visit was opportune. I'd just published the paper in the *New England Journal of Medicine* showing that cytomegalovirus (CMV) was a sexually transmitted infection, a concept not accepted initially as you've heard.

During my visit, I met Dr. Jackson, and we had kinship. His keen and critical mind and his sense of humor drew me in. I don't know what he saw in me. But later in the interview, he was serious and intense. "OK, Jordan, you can come into the lab. Barbara and I will help you. But you sink or swim on your own merits. We're tired of MDs coming around for advice, expecting us to help them with their research, and then, we get nothing in return. They use us. Now I admit, we've never had a physician who actually wanted to work in the lab. But don't think Barbara and I will do your experiments for you while you run around the hospital seeing patients, making twice the money we do."

He'd be a taskmaster, and I'd give in to his track record. After all, excellence was excellence. What else was there?

———

After rounds, I came back to the Jackson laboratory. Something festive was going on. As I walked down the hall, Steven called out. "Jordan! Come down here. We're having a party in your honor. Any excuse for a party!"

As I came into the conference room, the laboratory staff was there; Era, the chief cook and bottle washer, Vivian and Jennifer, the senior technicians, John and Kelly, the postdoctoral fellows, Howard, a professor on sabbatical from Edinburgh, and, of course, Barbara Covington. Bottles of wine, at least two of which were empty, stood on the table. Jackson put his hand on my shoulder. "After you interviewed for a job here, Jordan, I took a poll among the five senior lab members as to the likelihood of you succeeding. The results were 3 to 2 in favor. After you were here for a year, they were to 5-0. But then, when we found out you were getting a divorce, it went to 2-3. Some figured you'd bolt for private practice. Today, after your work was accepted for presentation at the herpes virus workshop at Harvard, we say again 5-0! Congratulations!"

After the festivities, Jackson called me into his office. "You've got a little over a month to pull this presentation together. We can have as many rehearsals as you like, but I don't think you'll need many. Just remember the cardinal rule of this laboratory when giving a paper. Don't exaggerate the experimental results. The simplest, not the most profound, explanation is likely. Don't try to make too much of the data. Then, review carefully the weaknesses in your results. Bring them up yourself before someone else can in the question and answer period that follows. It's critical that the paper be given in a balanced way. In other words, be your own worst enemy."

I didn't tell Steven I'd had little trouble lately being my own worst enemy.

CHAPTER 15

HECTIC FEVERS

Sutton's Law Goes Awry

I had clinic the next morning. None of the patients was as ill as the medical student sitting next to me writing in a chart. He was huge, six-feet-six-inches tall and more than two hundred and eighty pounds I'd guess. Sweat was all over his the face, and his white jacket was soaked. He was pallid, obviously anemic. I reached for his hand. "Hi. I'm Colin Jordan from infectious diseases. Are you OK? You don't look well."

"Jonathan Filtzer. Yes, I know you. You gave the virus lectures to our class two years ago with Dr. Jackson. Thanks for your concern. I'm having fevers and losing weight. I have an appointment in Student Health this afternoon."

Later that day, during rounds, Dr. Charles Bierman paged me. "Sorry to bother you, Colin. I know you're on the consult service, and you're busy. I'm seeing a medical student I think you're familiar with, Jon Filtzer. I just examined him, and he looks terrible! Some of his lab work is back. He's profoundly anemic with a hemoglobin level of 7.7 grams. His white blood cell count is over 60,000. And his sedimentation rate is 110. I'm afraid he has some horrendous infection I'll never diagnose. Can see him this week? I hate taking care of medical students. It's too stressful, you know, those constant calls from the damned Dean's Office."

"I can see him tomorrow, Charlie."

"Oh, bless you! Did you know he was an All-American defensive tackle at Stanford? They upset Ohio State in the Rose Bowl three years ago. He was the most valuable player. I remember watching him on T.V. He was a brute, an animal."

———

I didn't know we were setting off on a torturous journey. With this history, Jonathan had us on the hunt the next day in clinic. He'd been to Northern California, spending a week with his family. Driving down the coast back to Los Angeles, sudden abdominal pain overcame him in the epigastric area, just below the sternum. He pulled over on the road and "curled up in a ball" in his car. He fell asleep for two to three hours and woke up drenched in sweat. From then on, over the last three months, he'd had fever daily, often as high as 104 degrees. The abdominal pain never came back, but he weakened and continued to sweat profusely.

"You kept working on the wards all that time without seeking help? Were you in denial?"

"I guess so, Dr. Jordan. I've never been sick a day in my life."

On examining him, I found surprisingly little. The mucous membranes of his eyes and oral cavity were exceedingly pale, as were his fingernails. But I already knew he was anemic. I found nothing when I examined his abdomen where I expected to find the key to his illness. I left the room while Jonathan dressed. Everything he'd described had a straightforward explanation. He'd perforated a duodenal peptic ulcer driving back to Los Angeles, which would explain the sudden pain. The fever and anemia that followed were due to an abscess in his upper abdomen, now walled off by a thick membrane.

The hypothesis didn't set quite right. I suspected a disease more cryptic where the abdominal pain was a "red herring," but what was it? A lymphoma? A collagen-vascular disease like lupus or polyarteritis? Although it was his initial complaint, the pain had never come back. Throughout the training of a physician, the professors emphasized that "common things are common." Obviously then, a perforated duodenal ulcer explained it all. The axiom went, "when you hear hoof-beats coming up behind you, think horses, not zebras." But I worried about zebras because so few others did, and someone in the jungle had to be on the lookout. Zebras were more interesting; ah yes, a daunting and sometimes grueling check on a doctor's mettle. Mine was about to be tested.

I arranged Jonathan's admission to the internal medicine ward. I honed my wiles, expecting to negotiate or use diplomacy with the attending physician. I was surprised when Dr. Helen Skogsrud said, "Whatever you want to do is fine, Colin."

Then I realized I'd been "snookered." She didn't want anything to do with those calls and questions from the "damned Dean's Office" either. As I was dictating my clinic notes, I remembered more of my conversation with Filtzer. "Jonathan, you're Jewish right?"

"Yes."

"Is there any Sephardic background in your family?"

"No. Strictly Ashkenazi as far as I know."

"Do you mind asking your parents?"I'd brought it up because over 250,000 Sephardic Jews lived in California. Their ancestors had been driven out of Spain during the Inquisition, and many had migrated to North Africa. The Sephardic Jews I knew in Los Angeles were remarkable people who spoke Spanish, French, Hebrew, Arabic, and English.

The potential significance of a Sephardic background had to do with a genetic disorder called Familial Mediterranean Fever. Usually, but not always, it starts out in childhood. Sudden bouts of fever and abdominal or chest pain are its *modus operandi*. Inflammation of the membranes that line the abdominal cavity and the lungs occur repeatedly. Before the eventual diagnosis, numerous unnecessary surgical procedures, in a search for abscesses or perforated abdominal organs, have typically been done. Scars reflecting that history are conspicuous on physical examination. Ironically, a cheap old-fashioned drug called colchicine, used for over a century to manage gout, treated acute episodes and prevented recurrent attacks. A piece of cake if the doctor recognized the disease.

———

The following day, just before consultation rounds, I went to see him. Jonathan was in good spirits, relieved to be in custody I thought. Leaving the room, I ran into Dr. Skogsrud. "I just found out, Colin, that the gallium scan on Filtzer shows a collection of fluid behind the duodenum consistent with an abscess. The radiologists say there's no other explanation for the findings. Sounds like he needs a surgical exploration, huh? The strange thing, though, is that the CAT scan wasn't nearly so clear cut."

"These gallium scans are new, Helen. Whenever a new test comes out, the radiologists sing its praises based on the journals they read. But they never want a follow-up on an actual patient with a positive scan. Have you ever had a radiologist call you and ask: 'By the way, what did that fluid collection turn out to be in Mr. Jones?' I haven't. Let me know when you get the call."

"I agree. But where do we go from here?"

I was relieved to hear her ask. Technically, as the attending physician, she could block any recommendations I had if she were inclined. But then, maybe I'd been "snookered" again. "Helen, let me check in with the radiologists. I'll call you later."

I didn't want to talk to the radiologists. I knew what they'd say, though I'd review the scans. I was buying time to collect my thoughts before we rushed to judgment. What didn't I like about this? The white blood cell count was too high for an intra-abdominal abscess. A normal white blood count was between 4,500 and 11,000. Usually, with an infection in the abdomen, it was typically 20-30,000, maybe 35,000. Jonathan's was now over 80,000. To me, it was a "leukemoid" reaction. I asked Helen to order a bone-marrow examination to make sure the problem wasn't leukemia, and she did. Leukemoid responses often signaled an adverse reaction to a drug or systemic inflammation not due to infection, but caused by a malignant tumor or collagen disease like lupus or another rheumatic disorder. I wanted to avoid surgery. My thoughts now seemed paradoxical, recalling the "Leukemia, my ass" episode with Senora Cisneros when I'd had a tantrum about getting surgery done sooner than later. Now I was dragging my feet.

I called Helen back. "Why don't we ask Bill Longacre to see Jonathan? He's a renowned abdominal surgeon and chairman of the department of surgery. He has mature judgment with conservative leanings when it comes to operating. I'd value his take."

"Do you mind calling him? I'm new here, and I'm not comfortable calling someone like that. By the way, a Dr. Harvey Williams, who I understand is the Associate Dean of Students, has been paging me about Filtzer. He's rude and obnoxious. Can you help me out with him too?"

Now I knew for sure I'd been "snookered." Harvey Williams paged me. "Why is it every damned time I have trouble with a medical student, you're in the thick of it, Jordan? Just like the last one, Barbara Engstrom, the United Film Studios Scholar. You'd better get to the bottom of it with Filtzer ASAP. He's likely the top student graduating this year."

Snookered and worried with no idea what was wrong with Jonathan, I slumped in a chair. I'd had enough of this mediocre phony with Harvard and Yale bullshit on his walls. Maybe my reaction said more about me than him. "Harvey, for Christ's sake, I count two medical students. (I guess he hadn't heard about Paul Webb). Would you be so worked up if Jonathan was at the bottom of his class? What the hell do you think we're doing outside your silly world? Maybe you should read a textbook and get up to date. Or take a continuing medical education course offered by the University. You can review the brochures your office sends out! When we have a diagnosis on Jonathan, you won't hear shit from me." We were done. *Soit. So be it.* We'd been done for years.

———

After he'd seen Jonathan, Bill Longacre paged me. "I went over him with a fine-toothed comb. He most likely has a perforated duodenal ulcer with a walled-off abscess in the lesser sac. I think he needs an abdominal exploration."

"OK, Bill. I think we have to operate. We can't *not* operate and miss an abscess."

You had to drain an abscess; surgeons and infectious disease specialists agreed. Antibiotic therapy didn't work because the organisms within were too numerous, and drugs penetrated poorly into the deepest portions of the abscess. Treatment with antibiotics was merely an adjunct to the cure, which was thorough drainage, just as it was before antibiotics were discovered.

"Let's just hope it is an abscess," I thought. "After all, everything fits doesn't it?"

Dr. Longacre called the next afternoon. "You know, Colin, it's the damnedest case I've ever seen or not seen, maybe I should say. He had nothing in his belly! The duodenum looked perfectly normal with no abscess or even inflammation in the vicinity. The pancreas was normal. I have no idea what the hell caused the abdominal pain. Or the high white cell count. Or the positive scan. Or the anemia! Humbling, I have to say."

"Bill, thank you. We needed to know. I feel sheepish now, dragging you into it. Does Jonathan know nothing was found?"

"No. He's coming out of anesthesia about now. My residents will tell him. Don't worry about dragging me in. How else do we learn?"

I wasn't surprised. But now, with the 20:20 wisdom of hindsight, we at least knew Jonathan didn't have an abscess. I didn't want to hear the next question. "Where do we go from here?" No, the damned question was "what do *you* do next?" I'd shot the only arrow in my quiver, and I'd missed.

As lead perpetrator in the debacle, I wanted to be the first to see him. When I got to the recovery room, he was alert and eager. He tried to sit up on the gurney, but the abdominal pain at the surgical site overcame even his massively muscled frame. Reclining reluctantly and grimacing, he gave me "two thumbs up" and asked, as you would expect of an exceptional medical student, ignoring what should have subdued him. "So, what did we find?"

"Jonathan, we didn't find anything; no abscess and no evidence of inflammation."

Silence, tears, and then rage. He banged his fists into the bedding and screamed. "Damn it, Dr. Jordan! I believed everything you told me! You're supposed to be a brilliant diagnostician. You're a phony! I should *never* have listened to you. You have no business taking care of anybody!"

"Maybe that's true. I know your pain, my massive friend, and I love you," I thought. "But we're not done. Give me time. I'll make it right. I usually do."

I knew if Jonathan could've ignored the pain long enough to rise from his bed, he'd have thrown his doctor through the window, all five-feet-eight-inches and one-hundred-fifty-pounds of him.

———

Weeks passed. The patient and his physician made their peace. Jonathan's symptoms started to change. The fever came on less often but higher in degree with teeth-chattering chills lasting several hours. I gave in to the solitude that comes on when you struggle with a patient with thorns all over him, and you have no one to call for help. I longed to be a doctor in Riverside, California so I could send him to Mecca for an expert opinion. Dig deeper, damn it. What are you're missing? Don't let Hugh Cummings down, the toothless veteran in Omaha who taught you how to do a "circ" time. He'd taught me more than that, and I hope he rests in peace.

"This won't go on forever will it without a sign, a breakthrough?" The brilliant black and white stripes on this magnificent zebra had slid to murky gray. Here we were again, medical practice gone murky, murkier than ever. I had no diagnosis in sight or in mind. With nothing on my list, I thought the unthinkable. I might lose him. Come on, dig in! What the hell is the matter with him? I prayed the "tincture of time" would save us; it had never failed me.

On occasion, he'd call to complain about a rash. "Meet me in that outside eating area behind the cafeteria, and we'll have a look at it." Each time we met, the rash was gone. Later on, after several transient rashes I didn't see, Jonathan called about a red, sore left ankle. When I saw him in the emergency room, fierce heat and swelling were all over the joint.

"Where had I read about this? High fevers, transient rashes, swollen joints, profound anemia, and white blood cell counts to the sky?" In time, I remembered. A colleague at the National Institutes of Health had recently published a paper on a disease of childhood coming on in young adults. In children, it was called "Still's Disease" or juvenile rheumatoid arthritis. It wasn't an infection or at least not an infection anyone knew the cause of. Typically, the illness began with high fever and fleeting ("evanescent") rashes, and, often many weeks to months later, eventually declared itself with arthritis. But the test for the rheumatoid arthritis seen in adults was always negative. In fact, there was no test for "Still's Disease;" the diagnosis rested on its "characteristic clinical and laboratory features," perverse as they were, coming in whatever sequence they liked to torment patients and doctors. So, in a sense, "juvenile rheumatoid arthritis" was a misnomer. The childhood disease and adult rheumatoid arthritis were probably not related.

Once again, what looked like a straightforward infection was something else causing high white blood counts, incapacitating fevers, rigorous chills, fleeting rashes, and eventually arthritis. In the end, the physician had to be an internist first and a sub-specialist second. Imagine that.

I started Jonathan on high doses of aspirin, up to sixteen adult-sized tablets a day. As I did more often than I liked, I was practicing "seat of the pants medicine." I had no idea what caused adult Still's Disease or how to treat it. His symptoms improved dramatically at first. The

M. COLIN JORDAN

fevers disappeared, his anemia resolved, and the rashes ceased. Weeks later, despite the aspirin, the symptoms returned, and he required a six month course of prednisone which is a corticosteroid and a drug I detest because of its horrific side effects.

Nearly a year later in June, I attended the graduation ceremony to see two medical students I loved receive their degrees as Doctors of Medicine. Often I was perplexed by the choices medical students made for their training; many chose a field I knew would leave them unfulfilled. Today, it wasn't the case, and I took pride in the influence I'd had on their careers and their lives. They were as good as it got, two of the finest young people medicine had to offer. Jonathan Filtzer would return to Northern California for a year of internal medicine prior to his ophthalmology residency at Stanford. Harvey William's prediction was right. Jonathan graduated as the number one student in the class. Paul Webb, son of a wine merchant in the San Fernando Valley, would go to the University of Washington for three years training in internal medicine and three in infectious diseases, anticipating an academic career in research and patient care. I'd told him all about the University, and I'd even called the 'Dorf to fill him in about Paul.

The three of us shared hearty rounds of hugs and handshakes. They both knew I loved them, but that probably wasn't on their minds. During the ceremony, I mused in pain as well. Where was their classmate, Barbara Engstrom?

I wasn't quite done with Jonathan. At Christmas, he sent me a card to say that he'd had a second abdominal surgery. His bowel was obstructed as a complication of the first operation. At times after abdominal surgery, thick bands of scar tissue called "adhesions" develop. Typically, they block bowel function, disabling the patient with abdominal pain and severe bloating. Surgery is usually needed again. I was crestfallen, feeling like the captain of a ship called "The USS Misadventure." Fortunately for both of us, the second surgery was the end of it as I learned every Christmas for the next ten years.

204

CHAPTER 16

WHEN PATIENTS ABUSE DOCTORS

Now that you've heard, not for the first or last time, how doctors abuse patients through happenstance, incompetence, or greed, it seems only fair to turn the question around. Do patients abuse doctors? Of course they do, though they'd never admit it either. They lie to us, deceive us, and lead us down blind alleys. Maybe the most common goal is to get narcotics for vague aches and pains. The doctor never knows how much pain a patient actually has. They have us over a barrel. Maybe it's to get the attention of the doctor, a spouse, a parent, or even a child. "You have no idea how much I'm suffering or how much I've suffered because of you," the patient says without saying it. "I'll damned sure make you aware of it now."

I'm not a psychiatrist, as you know, and I have no special training in the matter. But I have experience. Although I'd learned as an intern that patients took advantage of us to get narcotics, no one made it clearer than a man who came by ambulance on a night in winter to the Seattle VA. He showed up with the snow flurries in crisis mode; the lights flashing, and the sirens blaring. The ambulance attendant said when I met him outside. "I think he's having an MI (a myocardial infarction or coronary attack), Doc. Let's get him inside pronto."

Ernie Musher was a fifty year-old who told me he'd had an MI in San Francisco five years ago. I had no reason to doubt him. After the physical exam, I did an electrocardiogram (an EKG). He had "Q" waves in leads II, III, and AVF, consistent with a previous MI in the lower part of the left ventricle. He didn't have the S-T segment elevations typical of a fresh

MI, but it was well known that someone with a previous attack might not have them. The story came from his gut.

"I've been having angina, Doc, the last month. When I try to walk up stairs, it comes on just about every time. Or sometimes on level ground if it's cold outside. I don't dare have sex anymore. I get that damned squeezing sensation under my sternum." His right hand made a fist, and he had a look in his eye that got my attention, the look of a man who'd been there and knew of what he spoke. Whenever I saw that look, shivers shot up my spine, the look of a man who knew he might die at any moment.

"All I can do is stop to rest and slip a nitro (nitroglycerin) under my tongue. After about five minutes, I'm good to go again, hoping it won't come back anytime soon. I try to take as little nitro as possible. I don't like drugs. They scare me. Funny though, the pain doesn't radiate down my left arm like it did when I had the MI."

He had a degree in architecture from the University of California, Berkeley. Ernie lived in Seattle though he traveled a lot for his job. He had been seen in the ER at the VA hospital in Boise, Idaho last week, he said. They admitted him for three days, and blood tests ruled out an MI.

"Ernie, I'm going to admit you. I don't see anything acute on your EKG but, as you know, they're not always reliable in a situation like this."

"OK, Doctor, if you insist. But I'd rather go home. I hate hospitals."

I admitted him to the coronary care unit where he needed morphine to control his chest pain. I can't claim I doubted his story, but still I looked into it. Believe your patient but verify. The next day I called the Boise VA and spoke to the resident who'd been on his case. A Dr. Melman said. "Yeah, he gave me the same story except that he'd recently been at the Minneapolis VA. I called them just like you called me today. He stayed three days, but signed out against medical advice when they stopped his morphine. A resident gave me the same story I'm giving you. The guy is a morphine seeker. His medical records are always three VA Hospitals behind. Those Q waves on his EKG are pretty damned impressive aren't they? And then, he has the story to go with them. I had no idea he was scamming me. I was kind of disappointed that he hadn't actually had an MI. Or maybe I was just disappointed in myself."

"Yeah, the Q waves sure as hell are. And he has that look in his eye. Here's my beeper number if you have any follow-up when you get the records from Minneapolis."

I went up to the coronary care unit to see him the next morning. When he wasn't in bed number six, I asked the resident. "Where's Mr. Musher? Has he gone somewhere for a test?"

"No, he didn't have any tests scheduled this morning. I have no idea where he is."

He was gone, never to be seen again. At least, we'd cut his drug holiday short, maybe made it tough on him. I looked through his chart. He'd gotten four large doses of morphine, and his blood work had just come back; he hadn't had another MI. A few days later, I received a slew of records from six different VA hospitals. The story was always the same, and he'd been doing this at least three years. Maybe when we get electronic records, this kind of abuse will stop.

Ernie Musher had Munchausen's Syndrome, a factitious illness named after an eighteenth century German army officer (Baron von Munchausen) who loved to boast about and exaggerate his military exploits. Typically, the patients fabricate symptoms with a need to be seen as ill, deriving the secondary benefits of being cared for and cared about. Many all too willingly undergo numerous medical tests or surgical procedures. In other words, they're professional patients, but dishonest about it. Some, like Mr. Musher, have objective evidence of an abnormality, in his case the abnormal EKG. A physician had to take his complaints seriously, and he knew it. Not all of the patients, though, are drug seekers, rather more likely, seekers of affection and validation.

———

Donna Wilson was a twenty-six-year-old African-American who'd acquired HIV from a former boyfriend who was an intravenous heroin user. I'd picked her up as a patient when a colleague left the University about six months ago. The only symptom she had related to her HIV infection was burning and stinging pain in her lower legs and feet, HIV peripheral neuropathy. She'd never had an opportunistic infection. My colleague had started her on Tylenol #3 (acetaminophen with codeine) for the neuropathic pain. It was a commonly abused drug.

I gave Donna sixty tablets every two weeks. She was supposed to take a maximum of four a day, less if possible. It was never possible. She had a caregiver funded by the AIDS program established by the State. The role of the caregiver was to provide emotional support, to get the patient to clinic, to help her get medications, and so on. The program meant well but was ripe for abuse. Her caregiver, LaVonne, was a far bigger problem than Donna. Like clockwork, she'd call ten days after the last prescription, demanding a renewal. The reasons varied though they often recycled. "Donna's going out of town for a couple of weeks."

"Do you remember last time Donna went out of town? Well, she left her meds in the motel room."

"The neuropathy has been much worse than usual the last two weeks."

"Her sister stole the meds."

LaVonne and I had a number of heated conversations on the phone. We didn't see eye to eye; nor would we ever. Most often, I'd compromise and acquiesce to half the number of pills demanded, not wanting to leave Donna in the lurch. In clinic visits, I'd exhort her to try to use less medication and to make sure that the pills lasted the two weeks. I suggested that she try taking ibuprofen or some other non-narcotic analgesic instead of or in addition to the Tylenol #3. I succeeded only every so often, judging from the frequency of phone calls from LaVonne. She could be nasty on the phone. At one point, I threatened to contact the state to have her replaced as Donna's caregiver. That held her off for a couple of weeks.

In 1984, I decided to leave Los Angeles to take a position at the University of Minnesota as chief of infectious diseases. I sent out a letter to my patients, making arrangements to refer them to a new physician. On her last appointment, Donna said she had a confession to make and burst into tears. "I feel terrible about this, Doctor. You've been so kind in your care of me. I took the Tylenol #3 for about a week when it was first prescribed. I didn't help the neuropathy any. It made me nauseated and constipated. I haven't been taking it for over a year and a half. It's LaVonne who uses it like candy. I hope you can forgive me. Good luck in your new position in Minnesota. I hear it's a beautiful state, but the weather ain't so great."

Abby Abramson was a delicate little flower, thin as a rake. She'd been referred to the University Hospital for fever of unknown origin. The records from her private physician said she usually came to the office with a temperature of 104 degrees. She'd had an exhaustive work-up, and nothing had turned up.

After the resident presented Abby's case, we went in to see her. Talk about the eyes of a doe in the headlights. She was wounded, suffering in a private hell, maybe a hell of her own creation. Her temperature had been recorded that morning as 103 degrees. Once again, something didn't add up, imagine that. I said to the resident after we left Abby's room. "Something's not right here, Tim. Her pulse when we saw her was sixty-six which doesn't fit with a temperature of 103. Plus she doesn't feel hot. The physical exams and the lab work have always been normal at the outside clinic, and they are here too. Let's watch her when she takes her temperature. Have the nurses do them per rectum only, and ask the nurse to stay in the room but behind the curtain while the thermometer's in place."

The paper by Petersdorf and Beeson on "Fever of Unknown Origin" in 1960 had taught us that patients had numerous ways of bringing on their own "fever." It was yet another variant of the Munchausen Syndrome called "factitious fever." They could do it by putting the thermometer into their morning coffee or by injecting their own feces into an arm vein. I was reminded of a patient a few years ago when I'd found a tourniquet under the bedding as I examined him. I thought it had been left there by my sleep-deprived and brain-dead intern. But the patient had brought it in from home so that he could inject shit into a vein in his left antecubital fossa. The most adroit patients produced elevated temperatures by manipulating their rectal sphincters with friction sufficient to drive the reading on the thermometer through the roof.

In the afternoon, I went back to see Abby again. From her emaciated state and the way she picked at her food, I thought she had an eating disorder. Can a person with an eating disorder develop fever of unknown origin? Yes, of course. Anyone can.

"Why are you focusing on what I'm eating or not eating, doctor? The problem is that I'm having fevers, and no one can find the cause. I'm a mystery case, it's plain to see. I'm not going to answer any more of your dumb questions about my family, my boyfriend, or my job. Just get going on *your* job and find out why I'm having these damned fevers."

The next morning the head nurse hiding behind a curtain caught Abby pulling the thermometer out of her rectum, sticking it into a cup of coffee for thirty seconds or so, and then back into her rectum. That afternoon, Tim and I went in to see her. I said, "Abby, I think we know why you're having these high temperature readings."

"Oh good, we're finally getting somewhere."

"It's because you're inserting the thermometer into your coffee cup. The head nurse saw you do it this morning."

She started to cry. I stood up from my chair and put my arm around her. After about twenty seconds, she threw my arm aside and screamed at me. "Don't put your arm around me, you phony bastard! That's the first time I've ever done that with a thermometer. I was afraid the fevers would go away, and no one would do anything. That's the way it's always been; no one takes me seriously, just like you haven't. Well, that's your problem, not mine!"

She continued to cry. I didn't say anything for a few minutes.

"Abby, we've asked one of our staff psychiatrists to see you. Her name is Dr. Goldberg. She's very good, the best we have."

"They've pulled this shit on me before. I don't want to see a shrink. Give me the fucking paperwork to sign out against medical advice, and I'll do so gladly."

"We can do that, Abby, but please honor a request from me."

"What's that?"

"At least meet Laurie Goldberg before you go."

"OK, if it'll get me out of here."

Two months later, I was on the psych ward seeing a Vietnamese man admitted with profound depression. He had a positive skin test for tuberculosis and an abnormal chest x-ray; the team wanted advice. As I was writing my note, I noticed Abby Abramson's chart in the rack. She'd agreed to be admitted by Dr. Goldberg for treatment of anorexia nervosa. The chart didn't say much about "fever" except for a brief mention in the "Past Medical History." Laurie Goldberg, thank you. You *are* the best we have.

———

Maybe my take on it is too harsh; patients don't "abuse" doctors as much as they manipulate them. I first became aware of it as a third-year medical student. So, here I was brand new with a patient to see. Before then, the only patients I'd seen were in the physical diagnosis course. I'd never done a complete history and physical examination on a patient I was responsible for. Mary Harper was ready for me.

The best part of it was that my first attending physician, Dr. James Mueller, was said to have the finest bedside manner in the department of internal medicine. As it turned out, maybe it was good that he knew Mary from a previous encounter, but, then again, maybe not.

She was a handful. She was morbidly obese, and she didn't stop talking. During the "review of systems," she answered every question with an array of complaints. After twenty minutes, I hadn't gotten through the ears, eyes, nose, and throat. At this rate, I'd never finish before attending rounds with Dr. Mueller. Her thyroid was a concern. It crossed my mind that she blamed her obesity on low thyroid function, but her thyroid tests had always been normal. Still, a physician had started her on thyroid hormone a few years back, a common practice in heavy women then, and I hated the paternalism it took to do it.

"So, Dr. Mueller, I spent over an hour with her and didn't get to the physical exam. I'm sorry. I'll go back and examine her after rounds."

"I'm not surprised. Good luck there."

"What do you mean?"

"She's so fat you can't do a meaningful exam. You can't even get a decent x-ray. People need to know they can get so fat we can't take care of them."

I was getting a sense that the two of them had a history I wouldn't get beyond. I finished my presentation to Dr. Mueller the next day. "So, what do you think?" He asked.

"I had a hard time pulling it together in a way I could live with. I think her problems are functional with no physical basis, but we need to run some tests."

"Yes, I agree. Do you know what tests you want?"

"I wrote them down," I said, handing him a list.

"All this is reasonable. Go ahead and order the tests, and I'll see her with you in the morning."

It wasn't quite so simple. The blood drawing tech called me over to the nurses' station. "Mrs. Harper is so fat I can't find a vein in either arm. Can you do a femoral stick?" She wanted me to get blood out of a vein in Mary's groin. I asked a resident if he could do it for me. "No, I won't, but I'll show you how. We call it 'see one, do one, teach one.' First, you find the pulse of the femoral artery, and then you go with your needle about an inch medial to it. If you go laterally, you're going to hit the femoral nerve. That's not good. The patient will never forgive you. Let's go see her."

The next morning I was back in Mary's room to say that the tests were normal and that Dr. Mueller would be in shortly. "I don't look forward to him. That man doesn't like me."

"Nonsense, Mary. He's wonderful with patients. But take a bit of advice. When he starts to ask, don't claim to have every symptom in the book. Nothing ticks doctors off more than that. He won't believe you. Try to focus on what bothers you most."

"Thanks for you counsel, Doctor."

Was she being sarcastic because I wasn't yet a doctor, and I'd presumed to lecture her? Later on, it was obvious that I'd done her no good. While Mueller was in the room, the clock radio went off, just as it had been set. The voice came on when it was time. Trouble was brewing.

As Mueller stood there listening to a litany of complaints, he got more agitated by the minute, shifting his weight from one foot to the other. Then, his ears went red followed by the back of his neck. After about twenty minutes more than I expected him to tolerate, he interrupted and asked. "Mary, you know what you need?"

"No. What's that Dr. Mueller?"

"A swift kick in the ass."

With that, he turned and left the room, and I was there to pick up the pieces. Mary burst into tears. About an hour later, the ward clerk came in to say she'd been discharged by Dr. Mueller. She burst into tears again.

CHAPTER 17

READY FOR HARVARD

As my attending stint came to an end, I started work on the presentation for the International Herpes Virus Workshop. I'd been blessed with a research technician who did my experiments while I stumbled around the hospital trying to do the right thing. During those gaps when I was rarely in the lab, we'd meet two or three times a week to review data and plan experiments. "You've done beautiful job, Jenny. And it's all working for a change."

"Yeah!" she said in her extroverted way, raising a fist in the air. "You should go away more often."

"Maybe so, smart ass! Seriously, the data are great, and they couldn't come at a better time with the meeting just weeks away."

We'd bantered like this from the day I'd hired her. She was smart and ambitious, but not as tactful as she might have been. If you knew her kind heart, you weren't put off, but she didn't often show it. She drove an old Fiat she called "Giuseppe." The fan whirred on long after the ignition had been shut off, cooling the engine down I guess. Every time I saw the car, I was reminded of a job I had one summer in college working at a foreign car garage in Newport Beach. The mechanics hated to work on Italian cars because the nuts and bolts holding the engine or transmission together were neither American nor metric in caliber. Skinned knuckles and obscenities resulted. If an Italian car pulled up outside the garage for service, unless it was a Ferrari or Maserati, a sentry called out, "Fiat, mamma mia!"

The mechanics would stop working immediately, slide out from under vehicles, surround the owner of the Fiat, and sing, "M-I-C, K-E-Y, M-O-U-S-E! MICKEY MOUSE!" Fiat, of course, now owns a big chunk of Chrysler.

But today, Jenny had tears in her eyes. "I have to tell you something, Colin. I've been in L.A. for three years, most of it working for you. It's been good, but I need to get away. Life is nuts here, and. I miss my family. I want to go back to school for an advanced degree."

I'd hired her after she graduated in biology from the University of Minnesota. At the time, several medical schools had denied her application because her grade point average was just below the minimal qualification. She'd moved to Los Angeles to "find herself." Good luck on that one. "I'd like to keep you, Jenny. We could shoot for a promotion and a raise if you want to stay. Or do you want another crack at medical school? I can write a strong letter. Sometimes you have to be persistent, even stubborn. You're a better candidate now with your name on some publications. Not much to lose."

"Thank you," she said, blushing. "No medical school for me, seeing what you go through. I don't know what I was thinking back then. I'd like the science, but not the patient care."

———

I was tired now. The consultation service had a way of grinding you down, too many losses with way too much heartache; time for a white flag or maybe the towel thrown into the ring? You had clinic, other duties, and you were available seven days a week, twenty-hours a day. By the middle of the month, you were exhausted. But after the third week, new vigor from somewhere got you to the end of the month as if you could smell the finish line.

After leaving Jenny and the lab for the hospital, I got a page from Alicia Martinez, the manager in charge of patient billing for the Department of Internal Medicine. "I'm reviewing accounts receivable for the division of infectious diseases, Dr. Jordan. Your division is always weak in revenue compared to others, of course. You, in particular, are looking at a pace that won't generate enough money to cover your salary. I have a chance to sign up forty Los Angeles County Fire Department employees for routine physical exams. The Fire Department pays $150 for each exam, guaranteed. Plus, I figure, if you find something wrong with any of them, additional revenue will come in because they're all insured. I'd like you to sign up for it. The only downside I see is that you have to go to different fire stations around L.A. to do the exams."

I was appalled at her audacity. Alicia had no business deciding how revenue generated by infectious diseases should be allocated among the faculty members. Bill Hewitt had that job, bless him. Some years, certain physicians had a surplus, and it was shared in a "socialistic" manner with others who hadn't been as fortunate. Next year could a different story, but the procedure was always the same. Collectively, we came out just in the black with no bonuses unlike the rich Divisions in the Department (Cardiology, Pulmonary Medicine, Gastroenterology, and Kidney Diseases, the "procedure-based subspecialties"). We did the bottom fishing along with endocrinology, rheumatology, genetics, and general internal medicine ("the cognitive specialties" hardly had a procedure to do among them). Though we came to take a certain pride in our fate, the issue was still a source of chronic irritation.

I wasn't civil. "Alicia, additional revenue isn't likely because fire department employees, by screening, are healthy. No one will have findings that warrant further investigation. Today is my last day on the consultation service. We've had a busy month, bringing in a fair bit of money. Call Dr. Hewitt about this. I'm not doing it."

"But do any of these patients have sufficient insurance to pay for the services rendered, Dr. Jordan? That's what concerns me."

"Look, Alicia. I don't care about that. I see the patients I'm asked to see. I don't give a shit what insurance they have. They're our patients, aren't they? Are we supposed to turn our backs once we find out they don't have insurance? If you're so obsessed with this, why don't you look into what the Department and the Hospital can do to provide us more patients who *are* insured and stop hounding *us!* That's where the solution to the financial problems lies. I think you should get right on it."

Maybe Mack Hedges, the gastroenterologist with his colon scope, was right: "Several procedures in the morning, and I'm on the golf course by noon." Or did Harvey Williams have it right with his damage control and committee meetings? With a firm salary in hand from the Dean's Office, he probably never worried about a patient's health insurance because he never saw any patients.

I left for rounds telling myself that Alicia had a job to do, and she was doing it. But don't page me about shit like this when I'm on service. Send me a memo. No, don't send a memo. Call Dr. Hewitt and get his take on it.

That evening, my last on service, I hoped to escape with just a few pages. I'd seen a liver transplant patient with abscesses in her lungs and brain. I suspected a fungus called aspergillus, but other diagnoses were in the running. She needed surgery tonight, and the pathologist was to call with the results of the biopsy. The fungus was more or less untreatable in those days. Let's hope it's something else. The patient must have excellent health insurance or she wouldn't have had the transplant. Alicia Martinez would be pleased, but I wouldn't likely be happy.

I got the call about the liver transplant patient; the infection in her lungs and brain was due to aspergillus. The treatment then was a rat poison called amphotericin B, colloquially know as "ampho-terrible." We'd likely wipe her kidneys out using it. Nothing would change for decades. I went to bed despondent.

———

I spent all the next day in the lab. For some reason, the experiments were zipping along after a long drought typical of laboratory research. My work on CMV now focused on the latent infection, the infection transmitted by blood transfusion and organ transplantation, and the one that reactivated whenever a patient's immune system was suppressed by drugs or a disease such as AIDS. Organ transplantation transmitted the infection at an alarming rate; ninety-five percent in the case of liver transplantation. One of my colleagues had called CMV "the troll of transplantation" because it had become commonplace with a high death rate after an otherwise successful transplant.

To study the latent infection, and how it activated itself, I'd sought to develop a model in mice. I'd succeeded with Steven Jackson's support. When I gave the mice a small dose of the virus, they didn't become ill. Three months later, there was no trace of the virus in any organ. Yet, when I administered immunosuppressive medications, they all died within two weeks of widespread CMV infection. In other words, they acted just like people. Was that good or bad? We'd never been able to learn anything about latent CMV infection by studying people. Now, I hoped to identify the organs and cells that harbored the dormant virus, a subject nothing was known about. But did the experimental tools exist to exploit the model?

CHAPTER 18

HARVARD

The International Herpes Virus Workshop wasn't what I expected. I was surprised Steven Jackson hadn't warned me. Maybe he had a reason. The sessions started out well enough as I presented my research on the first morning of the three-day meeting. It was an honor to give a paper on the first day. I heard a number of laudatory comments about the work, and Steven seemed pleased. Subsequently, though, the scenario shifted as the tone of the meeting became vitriolic. I'd never seen such savagery at a scientific conference. The world only had room for five or six pre-eminent herpes virus laboratories it seemed, including Jackson's. Apparently, none of the directors could stand one another.

After each ten minute presentation, a professor from a competing laboratory rose in the audience and lambasted the speaker with personal attacks or undisguised innuendo.

"This is a song and dance like the one you gave us at the 1974 meeting. None of that work turned out to be right or even close."

"Sounds like the typical pap that comes out of your laboratory. I think you guys sit around in a think tank and then decide, 'Let's be the first to say this; it just might be true.' Try doing the proper experiments first."

"If you present experiments like these at an international meeting, your reputation will be unsalvageable if it isn't already."

Professors holding microphones made the remarks in the aisles of a sloping amphitheatre with over two thousand people in attendance. I was happy I'd given my paper. But I was too small a fish to warrant this kind of attention, at least for now. On the other hand, Steven Jackson

217

didn't miss a chance to have his say. Maybe, I had it all wrong, and it was just "jolly good" banter among cunning rivals.

On the final night of the conference, the organizers held a beer keg reception at the Harvard Faculty Center. I hadn't felt well all day, but decided to go. Boston was hot and muggy, and the congested Center had no air-conditioning. I took two sips of beer and was abruptly nauseated. Knowing I was in trouble, I bolted for the men's room like a full back carrying the football on a draw play. For some reason, the doors to the toilet stalls were locked. I turned instead to a urinal; it was just the right height if you were on your knees and needed to vomit.

Within moments, a Nobel Laureate who'd discovered CMV in 1954, wandered into the men's room. I was still on my knees, drenched in sweat. Fortunately, my retching had stopped, but I'm sure I looked a fright, pale and all. He said in a humble and congratulatory voice, "That was a wonderful paper you gave the other morning. We have a lot to learn about cytomegalovirus from your mouse model. And I think you're the man to do it."

"Thank you, Dr. Weller," I croaked, about to vomit again, hoping he wouldn't tarry.

———

Steven Jackson and I sat together on the flight back to Los Angeles. Sipping on his bourbon, he said. "Well, you did us proud. Thanks for the hard work. This is the lab's first foray into CMV. I'm glad you brought it to us."

"Thanks, Steve."

"What did you think of the meeting?"

"The nastiness shocked me. At clinical meetings, it's behind the back with a lot of snickering. Maybe it's good they get it out up front here."

"And you think nothing goes on behind the back at these meetings?"

"No, I didn't hear any of that. That professor from Zurich was something, wasn't he?"

"Yeah. He's a phony pompous ass, but he knows I'm on to him."

"How do you mean?"

"His career rests on feet of clay. I know it. He knows it. And he knows I know it."

CHAPTER 19

AIDS CHANGES ALL OF US

Michael S. Gottlieb, MD and six colleagues at UCLA Medical Center published a monumental paper in the *New England Journal of Medicine* on December 10, 1981. They reported the cases of four homosexual men with *Pneumocytis carinii* pneumonia, extensive candida or yeast infections, and multiple viral infections, including cytomegalovirus. Infections of this nature or severity didn't occur in people with normal immune systems. All four had severely diminished counts of CD4+ "helper" T-cells. We were about to learn that those cells were the quarterbacks or point guards of the human immune system and how we couldn't do without them.

Most of us scratched our heads and asked one another, "What the hell is going on?" Maybe our understanding of the immune system wasn't what it should have been. None of us had an inkling of the new era of devastation, misery, and death that was about to infect the human race. Gottlieb probably didn't either.

A dark and murky period followed. We wouldn't know the cause of this disaster until 1984, and we wouldn't have a blood test for it until 1985. In the meantime, we dutifully wrote and published reports on devastated, homosexual men and intravenous drug users. In the next round, it was the hemophiliacs, mostly children and young adults. Commercial companies were paying gay men, drug users, and prisoners to donate plasma for the production of the clotting factor hemophiliacs needed to stop or prevent bleeding. Six to ten thousand hemophiliacs in the United States died of AIDS over the next few years.

Before long, we were all at risk; homosexual men, injection drug users, heterosexual men and women, pregnant women and newborns, anyone who'd gotten a blood transfusion or an organ transplant, and health care workers. Doctors were now private detectives, sleazy voyeurs peering into bedrooms and bath houses, asking questions they didn't want answered. Holier-than-thou vigilantes hammered away for a while, clucking their tongue and wagging their finger, stigmatizing the guilty, but their message was soon passé. They shut up when AIDS went heterosexual, and they realized that any "red-blooded American boy" could catch it.

The landscape had forever changed and not only for infectious diseases doctors. Any health care worker who needed to draw blood or have contact with the bodily secretions of another person began to use "universal precautions." In other words, every patient was treated as if, risk factors admitted to or not, they might harbor an infection with HIV or the hepatitis B and C viruses.

Taking a medical history took on new twists. We were asking questions now that were unthinkable a year ago, and we were getting answers we'd never heard before, answers we didn't want to hear. Unpredictable scenarios were the norm.

Mike Mulcahy, tall, dark, and handsome, was a respected corporate attorney with a secret. He was admitted to the hospital with high fever, shortness of breath, and *Pneumocystis carinii* pneumonia. Prior to the AIDS epidemic, the organism was a cause of pneumonia in transplant patients or patients receiving prednisone to treat lupus and other diseases. The drug is a corticosteroid that suppresses the immune system when you have no choice but to suppress it because of the grief it's causing.

Once we had the results of the bronchoscopy and the blood work, I went to his room. He was more short of breath now. "Mike, you have pneumocystis pneumonia. And your T-cell helper count is very low. I'm afraid these results are consistent with a diagnosis of AIDS. I'm sorry."

He said nothing for a few minutes. Then, he blurted out "You're handing me a death sentence, aren't you?"

"No, not at all. We caught the pneumonia early, and we have drugs to treat it. But, we need to transfer you to the ICU to put you on a ventilator. You will make it."

"You doctors are so full of shit. You probably like my health insurance too, don't you? I have dollar signs all over my body, don't I? I'm not going to the ICU, and I refuse to be intubated."

"Mike, your health insurance has nothing to do with it. You don't understand. We can get you through this, and we will."

He *didn't* understand. The AIDS diagnosis had shocked him. As I left the room, I debated with myself. You don't go around intubating patients and putting them on ventilators against their will. If we could bring him back, what would he face, more opportunistic infections or cancers because of his weakened immune system? Someone out there might figure out what caused this hell before then. The debate was brief.

I paged the anesthesiologist on call and explained the situation. After she had seen Mike, she said. "Look, he's adamantly against intubation. I'm not sure we should be doing this."

"Yeah, I know. But he doesn't understand that he has a treatable infection. All he's thinking now is that he has fatal disease. He's in shock from the AIDS diagnosis. We'll get him through this. Just intubate him. If there is any fall out from the hospital ethics committee, I'll take the hit. Do you want me to sign something, Debbie?"

I could already hear the chairman of the hospital ethics committee asking. "So, doctor, can you explain to the committee how you had a patient intubated and put on a ventilator against his will with no signed consent form?" I'd already formulated my defense.

"What's more important, Mike Mulcahy's life or my hospital privileges?"

A week later, he was back on the ward and wanted to talk. He was bisexual. When he was traveling, he frequented gay bath houses. His wife didn't know or maybe she did. "So, what do I tell her?" He asked me.

"Well, you could tell her the truth."

"I can't do that. She has no idea. She'd flip out and leave me."

"I noticed that she didn't visit even when you were in the ICU. What have you told her so far?"

"Just that I had a bad pneumonia."

"Maybe she already knows or suspects something. Have you had unprotected sex with Nancy over the last few years?"

"Of course we have, depending on her cycle. I had no reason to have protected sex, did I?"

"From what you've told me, yes you did."

"Fuck you, doctor. She'll leave me if I tell her I have AIDS."

"You have to tell her. She's at risk too."

"Oh, Christ, I just can't do it."

"Do want me to do it?"

"No, I don't want that either."

"Mike, Nancy needs a helper T-cell count to see if she has AIDS. As your physician, I'll do my best to protect your confidentiality, but I can't do more. I can be there when you tell her if you like, or I will tell her. If you want to explain how you contracted AIDS, you can. I can't."

I don't know how it came about, but she left him a month later. When I brought Nancy in to clinic, she didn't want to talk about what she'd learned or why she'd left him though I'd left the door open. Fortunately, none of her tests indicated that she had AIDS. But we'd need to check her in six months and again in a year.

I took care of Mike for five years after the ventilator fiasco. He'd moved in with a gay lover by then, and Nancy was healthy and HIV-negative. Yes, we knew the cause of the disease and had a diagnostic test in 1985, a miracle at last. Sir Edward Jenner, a veteran of the foxholes and a miracle worker in his own time, smiled a wry smile down on us.

———

Other pieces of the puzzle began to fall into place. In 1982, I took care of Georgia Rosen, a sixty-two year-old dentist with a history of aortic stenosis due to a calcified bicuspid valve. The aortic valve normally has three cusps. When the valve has only two cusps from birth, it's prone to calcium deposits that gradually narrow the opening. After the onset of left-sided heart failure and fainting spells because of the obstruction and strain on her ventricle, Georgia had had a valve replacement in 1972. Her course was complicated by heavy bleeding into the chest, and she received eight units of blood to replace her losses.

Eleven years later, she showed up at the University Hospital with fever and lost vision in her left eye. She had AIDS with disseminated CMV infection involving the retina. Georgia had no risk factors other than the blood transfusions. We realized then that the incubation period from the time of infection to the development of overt AIDS, at least when it was acquired by blood transfusion, could be over a decade. In other words, we were dealing with a disease that came on as a consequence of an event, a blood transfusion or a sexual encounter, that happened years ago. We desperately needed a test to diagnose the infection before AIDS developed, and sooner than later. As noted, we had one in 1985, but it didn't help the patients we'd already lost.

———

By the time AIDS came along, we were used to dealing with suppressed immune systems from cancer chemotherapy and organ or bone marrow transplantation, but we weren't ready for this. The most striking aspect of AIDS from an infectious disease standpoint was how bizarre the opportunistic infections were, showing up in ways they never had before. What we were in for dawned on me when I saw my first cases of CMV in patients with AIDS. I knew what the virus could do, but I no longer had the full picture. CMV was known to cause retinitis occasionally in transplant recipients, but now it involved the eye as its organ of choice. AIDS patients never developed CMV pneumonia which had been its modus operandi in transplant patients. And the second most common manifestation of CMV in AIDS patients was in the gut, previously reported, but I'd never seen a case until now.

Pneumocystis went through a similar transformation. We knew the pneumonia well by then in transplant patients and cancer victims on chemotherapy. But now it was showing up with normal chest films, unheard of. And it no longer occurred with an abrupt onset. Patients were coming in with an indolent two or three week illness, and now they had lesions in the retina or abscesses in their spleens. *Pneumocystis carinii* occurring anywhere outside the lung was unheard of.

A bug in the same family as *Mycobacterium tuberculosis* (the cause of tuberculosis) called *Mycobacterium avium-intracellare*, a soil organism previously causing stubborn pneumonias in patients with chronic lung disease was now causing an aggressive form of blood poisoning with hectic fevers. Our world was upside down, and we needed to hone our coping skills. What was next and when would it stop? It still hasn't.

Fifth disease (erythema infectiosum) is one of six childhood illnesses characterized by fever and a diffuse rash. It's also called "slapped cheek disease" because of the typical eruption on both sides of a child's face. In 1983, the cause was found, parvovirus B19. Soon after, we learned about a symmetric arthritis in young women, many of whom had children in daycare where fifth disease was rampant. The arthritis in these mothers was caused by parvovirus B19 too.

The virus also caused rapid falls in the production of red blood cells in patients who had abnormal hemoglobin, such as those with sickle-cell disease. They developed aplastic crisis or pure red cell aplasia, a sudden profound anemia. Diagnosis of the infection relied upon the detection of a transient anti-viral macroglobulin antibody (immunoglobulin M or IgM) in the patient's blood. Patients with previous parvovirus B19 infection, now immune to the virus, had only anti-viral immunoglobulin G or IgG) in their blood. You might have suspected that this virus would do *something* bizarre in AIDS, but what would *something* be? We didn't find out until the early '90s.

Bill Halloran was a gay man I'd taken care of for about six months. On his second visit, I started him on the two drugs we had to treat HIV infection. Both were poisons that may have done more harm than good, zidovudine (AZT or Retrovir) and didanosine (ddI or Videx). Typical side effects were bone marrow suppression from zidovudine or pancreatitis and peripheral neuropathy from didanosine. They were all we had, or maybe they had us.

After he had been on therapy for a couple of months, I was called down to the ER to see Bill. On exam, he was pale as a ghost and profoundly anemic. When I'd started treating him, his blood hemoglobin concentration had been normal, around fourteen. Now it was five. He said to me. "I didn't know what was happening, Doc. Over a week or so, I felt weak all over, and I had no energy. All I wanted to do was sleep. When I looked at myself in the mirror this morning, the color in my face was gone."

At first, I thought it was a side effect of one of the drugs, most likely zidovudine. Though usually quite low after zidovudine toxicity, his white blood cell count was normal. We did a bone marrow examination and giant pronormoblasts typical of parvovirus B19 infection were seen. I knew about parvovirus B19 at the time and had ordered antibody tests for both IgM and IgG. Neither was positive, and the results didn't make sense. What we didn't know was that AIDS patients couldn't make antibodies against parvovirus. I guess the point guard of the immune system (the CD4+ helper T-lymphocyte) had never learned the plays.

Serendipity came to the rescue. A procedure for amplifying minute amounts of DNA into millions of copies had been described in 1987, the polymerase chain reaction or PCR. It revolutionized molecular biology, medical diagnosis in general, and management of HIV disease in particular.

When I ordered a PCR for parvovirus B19 on Bill's serum, he had over ten million copies of viral DNA in his blood. I treated him with human immunoglobulin G (IgG), a pooled preparation of immune globulin taken from thousands of donors. Statistically, it was likely to contain antibodies against parvovirus B 19 which by now we knew was a common infection in the general population. In other words, we gave him the antibodies the B-cells in his immune system, out of touch with the depleted helper T-lymphocytes, couldn't make for him. He had a dramatic recovery.

——

Infections kept coming at us in ways we hadn't seen or "heard of." But now, "unheard of" requests from patients and families came our way too. Clifford Dixon was a gay man, though you'd never have guessed it. By now, we'd gotten pretty good at telling who was a closeted gay man or one in denial, and Cliff wasn't one. He was "just gay, pure and simple" with a boyish joy about him when he told you. A dedicated young nurse practitioner, he died from his first AIDS-related infection, a brain abscess caused by toxoplasma, a protozoan parasite.

A few days later, his mother, a professor at the University, called me "to discuss a sensitive issue." She wanted me to say on his death certificate that Cliff had died of leukemia. "Barbara, I can't do that. I can't falsify a death certificate. It's a legal document."

"I don't want anyone in the family to know he was gay. His dad doesn't either."

"Did either of you have a problem with it?"

"No, we loved him. No one else knew. They wouldn't have accepted it."

"That's the trouble with AIDS, Barbara. Everybody wants the stigma swept under the rug. About five percent of the population is gay. Why not be open and get more people to accept it?"

"All well and good for you, Doctor, but you don't know my family."

Getting off my high horse, I said, "Barbara, AIDS isn't about homosexuality anymore. One of the world's best athletes, the tennis player Arthur Ashe, was just diagnosed with AIDS. He got it from blood transfusions. Heterosexuals are getting AIDS now, and many of them have no idea how. We'll make more progress if we refuse to stigmatize it. You don't need to explain to anyone how Cliff was infected. "

"Thank you, doctor. I don't agree, but at least you gave me an out."

Her voice was quaking now. "But then, Cliff wasn't your son, was he? Put AIDS on the certificate if you have to. My husband and I will deal with it. Thanks so much for your time."

We weren't done. Too many appointments went like this now, maybe my fault. I'd been on the defensive. As she rose to leave, I reached across the desk to give a hug. "Barbara, I loved Cliff. We all did. Tell his dad how much we grieve for his loss."

She sat down again and cried a while. I had only a vague notion of what she felt or thought. We'll need every ounce of wisdom the tincture of time can give to deal with this damned disease, to say nothing of what it did to those left behind.

————

The problem wasn't so much that we couldn't adjust to new pitches being thrown at us. We adapted as each bit of information came along. Still, we weren't ready for the problems about intimate relationship coming up.

Ernesto Montero was a forty year-old man from Mexico who'd become an American citizen in 1985. He held a supervisory position in a construction company and often worked out of town. One morning, he didn't show up on the site. Two of his co-workers went to look for him at the hotel. Ernesto was found comatose on the floor and admitted to a local hospital.

He turned out to have pneumococcal meningitis, an aggressive community-acquired infection with a death rate around thirty-five percent.

During the course of his evaluation, his physician noticed that Ernesto had a very low lymphocyte count in his blood. When his helper T-lymphocyte count came back, it was low at 180. A count below 200 was now considered diagnostic of AIDS by the Centers for Disease Control. An HIV antibody test was ordered and came back positive.

After his recovery and return home, Ernesto was referred to me in clinic. He denied any risk factors for HIV infection. When I asked whether he'd had any homosexual encounters, he hesitated before saying "no." I was a bit suspicious knowing that homosexuality was said to be unacceptable among Hispanics. Doctors were a suspicious and skeptical lot by then.

He had married for the first time about five years ago. His wife Cecilia had been married once before and was the widow of a man who died in Mexico of "a mysterious form of leukemia." Ernesto acquired two daughters when he married "CC" as he called her. I started the dance all too familiar now. "Does CC know about the AIDS diagnosis?"

"No, I didn't understand it myself until you explained it today. Does she need to know?"

"Yes, because the two of you have had unprotected sex. She could be infected. Do you feel comfortable telling her or do you want me to do it? We could bring her in to clinic."

"No, let me tell her. Just give me a chance, a few days."

After a week, I called him, and there was no answer. I called several times over the next few days, still no answer. I thought. "He wasn't able to do it or maybe they flew the coop."

A week later, after I'd finished morning clinic, I ran into the two of them in the lobby. He'd told her, and she was here for the test. When I filled out the lab slip, I noticed that CC's medical record number was older than Ernesto's. I looked up her record on the computer. She'd been referred to surgery clinic five years ago with swollen lymph nodes in her neck and armpits. A biopsy was performed. The immunological stains showed that she had virtually no helper T-cells in her nodes. No one had followed up on the results.

The HIV test on CC came back positive, and her CD4+ helper T-cell count was twenty, far below Ernesto's. She'd probably had the infection longer than he had. So, who'd given HIV to whom? And what was the "rare form of leukemia" her first husband had died of in Mexico? I tested the daughters, and, thank God, they were negative. I referred CC to a female colleague. By now, I'd learned not to take care of partners in a committed relationship if HIV was involved. One or both of them might be lying to you.